CARNAL
ACTS

CARNAL ACTS

Essays

NANCY MAIRS

Beacon Press
Boston

Beacon Press
25 Beacon Street
Boston, Massachusetts 02108-2892

Beacon Press books
are published under the auspices of
the Unitarian Universalist Association of Congregations.

The following essays have appeared previously: "Shape" in *Intro 13;* the "Hers" columns in the *New York Times;* "On Uttering the Unspeakable," written for the conference "Literary Women," Long Beach, California, February 1987, in the *Women's Review of Books* under the title "Speaking the Unspeakable"; "Faith and Loving in Las Vegas" in *The American Voice* and in *The Bread Loaf Anthology of Contemporary American Essays;* "Carnal Acts" in *TriQuarterly;* "Challenge: An Exploration" in *Tucson Lifestyle;* "Doing It the Hard Way" in *Kaleidoscope;* "I'm Afraid. I'm Afraid. I'm Afraid." and "Where I Never Dreamed I'd Go, and What I Did There" in *The American Voice;* an excerpt from "Good Enough Gifts" in *Working Mother.*

Excerpt from the essay "Stabat Mater" by Julia Kristeva, copyright © 1990 by Columbia University Press, New York. Used by permission.

Text design by Cassandra J. Papps

01 00 99 98 97 96   8 7 6 5 4 3 2 1

Library of Congress Cataloging-in-Publication Data

Mairs, Nancy, 1943–
    Carnal acts : essays / Nancy Mairs.
        p. cm.
    Originally published: New York, NY : HarperCollinsPublishers, c1990.
    ISBN 0-8070-7085-8 (paper)
    1. Mairs, Nancy, 1943– —Biography. 2. Women authors, American—20th
century—Biography.   3. Multiple sclerosis—Patients—United States—
Biography. 4. Women and literature—United States. I. Title.
    [PS3563.A386Z464 1996]
    814'.54—dc20   96–15131

for Anne and Matthew
best beloved blessings of my carnal acts

What is loving, for a woman, the same thing as writing. Laugh. Impossible. Flash on the unnameable, weaving of abstractions to be torn. Let a body venture at last out of its shelter, take a chance with meaning under a veil of words. WORD FLESH.

—Julia Kristeva,
"Stabat Mater"

Contents

But First,

A couple of years ago, I was granted what may be every writer's dearest wish: the chance to work at writing a book without the distraction of an outside job. I wasn't sure just what this writing life would entail. I'd never written a book on purpose before. But I gamely rented a casita at the edge of the barrios in downtown Tucson for a studio, set up my word processor on a cast-off dining room table, bought a statue of Our Lady of Guadalupe to put in the pointed niche above the fireplace, and sat down to begin. Alone here, without a telephone on which women could call offering to photograph my babies (who are twenty and twenty-four) or to exterminate my pests (except, alas, themselves), without a washing machine in which to agitate my husband's soiled socks, I would, I believed, devote several hours a day to the exercise—so long suppressed or distorted by the demands of children,

1

professors, students, and cats with plastic dinosaurs stuck in their guts—of my creativity.

I overestimated both my stamina and my self-discipline. For what seemed like years but was about four months, nothing much happened at all. Actually, in the sour judgment of one reviewer, nothing much ever happened. But in fact—haltingly and with a vaster amount of pain than I'd thought I could tolerate but also with richer satisfaction than I could have anticipated—I did finally write a book. And in the process I learned a fair amount about the life of a working writer, at least of *this* working writer.

One of the things I learned is that she may spend a lot of time *not* writing a book. A good bit of the time I lost was my own fault, of course. I can be a poor taskmistress, with myself as with anyone else who's worked for me, sympathetic and lenient when it comes to menstrual cramps and visitors from out of town. Even so, I get to my studio most days for about six hours. Once there, however, I'm apt to spend more time reading than writing. The truth is that I'll do *anything* rather than write, even read French phenomenology. Reading French phenomenology is, in fact, a particularly seductive activity, since, unable to understand a word of it (even in translation), I have to read every passage over again, thus filling a great many hours with what must be—by virtue of the incomprehensibility of the material—an intellectually virtuous pursuit. But even if I did nothing but twiddle my thumbs during the time I now spend reading, it turns out, I wouldn't be able to write for more than two to three hours. I simply don't have the physical endurance to prop my crippled form in front of the screen for longer. My fingers go every which way. Then I start feeling frustrated and weepy and whatever energy was directed at my task transforms into anger at my failing body. (As it has just now. I'm going home.)

(Next day.) But another reason for not writing a book, I learned, is that one gets busy writing something else. I don't think I'd realized that, if I gained any reputation at all, people would start asking me to write for their publications or, more daunting yet, to come and speak to them just as though I were one of those real writers whose readings and lectures I'd been attending for a good quarter of a century. I don't speak, however. At the thought of standing at the front of a room, even a small one, building from the jottings on a handful of three-by-five cards something even sensible, much less graceful and entertaining, I can't draw in enough breath to whisper my own name. I'm a *writer.* Whenever I accept an invitation to speak, then, I write an essay and, sheltered by a sheaf of printed pages, I can throw my voice to the back of quite a large ballroom.

As a consequence, in the course of writing a book on purpose, a memoir called *Remembering the Bone House,* I began to generate enough material for another book, quite different in structure and intent. An accidental book, should I call it? A collection of occasional pieces, their purpose and length and content often only partly my own choice, bound not, like *Bone House,* by the necessities of memory and desire but merely by the voice that, in response to some bidding, utters them. The drawback to such a collection is that it can't possibly cohere in the

3

ways that distinguish an intentional book. It's inevitably something of a mess.

In fact, I tried to make it more of a mess than it's turned out. With the exception of fragmentary or unfinished material, I had planned to include most of the public pieces I've written in the last five years, among them literary essays and reviews as well as more personal meditations and addresses to a variety of audiences, many of them involved in some capacity with the community of people who live with multiple sclerosis. For me, thinking about literature and thinking about life aren't separate, or even separable, acts. When my editor chucked more than a hundred pages on the grounds that they were too "academic," I was stung by the implicit message that the interest of publishers and audiences could be piqued only by part of me: the damaged part. I felt creepily like old what's-his-name, coming to and peering down and asking, "Where's the rest of me?"

But that's silly. I'm all here, in these pieces as in the ones excluded. A writer always writes with her whole being. And I think that the material that remains has kept what I see as the advantage of an "accidental" book. That is, it reveals the writer at work: the ideas she cherishes or repudiates; the jokes she likes best; the themes and images that draw her; and, if the pieces are arranged chronologically, the direction of her development. I am very aware, for instance, of the emergence in these writings of my body: that is, of a literal, physical constellation of events which, day after day, must be put on, and sometimes over, the line. It has assumed an experiential focus so powerful that, in the end, I have come to take the essays here, all together, as *Carnal Acts.*

"My body is going away," I began a poem seventeen years ago, shortly after learning that I had multiple sclerosis. And that must have seemed to me what was happening, as my muscles shrank and refused to do my bidding, as holes appeared in my vision, as I had to give up the hiking and camping and dancing I'd always enjoyed without question. Loss. Loss. Loss. But I was wrong to think of it, as the poem went on to say, as fading to the transparency of amber. It has, on the contrary, grown thicker and more opaque over time. It looms in my consciousness now as it never did when all my gestures were as thoughtless as yours perhaps still are. Pouring the glass of wine, raising it in a toast, putting it to your lips, you are perhaps lost in the eyes of your beloved or in the oaky crispness of your Chardonnay, depending on your priorities. I am trying to prevent my fingers from releasing the stem and dumping icy wine in my beloved's crotch.

What I am saying is that I must now *attend* my body—both in the sense of "fix the mind upon" and "watch over the working of" it—in ways that I never dreamed of and that you may still find foreign. As Edwin Kenney pointed out in a letter to the *New York Times Book Review* (January 14, 1990), "to be seriously ill, in itself, removes one from the general definition of ordinary experience." In that sense, the pieces in this book arise from, reflect upon, and try to illuminate "extraordinary" circumstances. No one is protected from such circumstances, however. In writing about my experience, I am, first of all, trying to make sense of it and to make it bearable for myself. But I am also trying to draw you into it, to carry

5

you along through it, so that whatever extraordinary circumstances you one day meet—and you will, because all creatures do—you will have, in some way, "been there" before. As you can see, I'm the sort of person who likes to meditate on maps before heading off into new territory. I also like to plan my wardrobe and anticipate in macabre detail every disaster that might befall a traveler, no matter how wary. Thus prepared, I can give myself over to the trip.

The reviewer I mentioned earlier excoriated me for, among a great many other things, suggesting in my preface alternate ways of reading *Remembering the Bone House.* Clearly, he knew the one true way of reading a book: beginning on page one and working his way painfully straight through. The product myself of the puritanical academic training that must have molded him, I too tend to read in dogged linear fashion, believing that skipping or skimming somehow constitutes cheating— cheating *who,* I'm not certain. I don't see why anyone else should adopt the same strategy, however; nor do I see why I shouldn't recommend other approaches. I know what's here, after all, and you don't; but you know, as I don't, what you prefer to read; and we should collaborate, it seems to me, in order to get for you as much pleasure as possible.

For this reason, I'd like to talk a little here about each of the pieces that follow, giving you a chance to pick and choose. I'd like to be able to say that there's something here for everybody, but of course I can't. I'm a woman with a particular set of characteristics: a white, middle-aged, middle-class, heterosexual, crippled feminist of a reclusive and rather bookish temperament, turned from New England Congregationalist to Roman Catholic social activist in the desert Southwest. Because I write as directly as possible out of my own experience, these traits inevitably shape my work. The best I can hope for is that there's something here for somebody, and that that somebody will sometimes turn out to be you.

I've begun this collection of essays with a short story, in part because, except for a couple of little lyrics early on, it represents my first public attempt to address the issues of embodiment forced on me, as both a practicing mother and a practicing artist, by multiple sclerosis. More important, however, it demonstrates something I learned from that attempt: that fiction was not going to enable me to do what I wanted to do with my material. Just what I wanted to do wasn't clear to me nearly ten years ago, when I wrote "Shape," but after I experienced the feeling of distance between myself and my narrator, who was not me in spite of the fact that I'd made her up and even included some autobiographical fragments, I knew I wanted to speak more plainly about my preoccupations.

Every piece of writing, whether "fictional" or "factual," entails the creation of a persona, of course: a mask. I am not the woman whose voice animates my essays. She's made up, too, constructed just as much out of language as Pamela, the narrator of "Shape," is. But I am more the woman of my essays than I am the woman of my fiction, because she and I share the same past. And so, understanding with greater clarity as I kept writing that I wanted to make sense of my own experience as it

7

illuminates human experience more generally, I turned to writing nonfiction. Rather than remove myself from my life, as I felt I was using fiction to do, I've tried to scribble myself deeper and deeper into it.

That was the attempt that motivated me in the six pieces I was invited to write for the "Hers" column of the *New York Times.* Having no journalistic experience, I found these a useful discipline, because they had to be short (about nine hundred words) and I had to write them in a hurry. But, because the choice of subject was entirely mine, they also provided me the chance to pin down and concentrate on several concerns that were currently preoccupying me.

Most rewarding of all, these columns generated direct, almost immediate responses: a lot of people read the *Times,* and a fair number of them talk back. Over the years, I've had many letters and even some telephone calls in response to my books, but these arrive sometimes years after I've finished writing. By contrast, the dozens of letters from *Times* readers—some of them funny and several downright unflattering—arrived while my thoughts were still so fresh that I felt almost engaged in dialogue. One called me a "female chauvinist sow." "If you are being given a chance to write the 'Hers' Column," said another, "try to write something worth reading." The ones I most treasure came from the members of an Adult Basic Education class in Brooklyn who were laboriously making the transition, attested by the letters themselves, from illiteracy to literacy.

Yet another correspondent practically wept with pity for my husband, with some reason, it turned out. The following year, a researcher for the "Oprah Winfrey" show came upon the piece on marriage-as-housework and invited George and me to appear on a program about communication in marriage. With the exception of our accommodations at the Nikko Hotel (where George ate—honest to God—raw tuna stomach with a raw quail egg broken into it and salmon blood, but I did not), this was one of the most disagreeable experiences we've ever shared. The approximately twenty-five minutes left after deleting the advertisements (as my sister did in videotaping), fragmented among at least seven commercial breaks, permitted only the most hasty and shallow remarks. These were dominated by a marriage therapist who had, in the limo on the way from the hotel to the studio, spoken of his ex-wife in the bitterest terms I've ever heard one human being use about another.

Afterward, we were immediately driven to the airport, where George flew back to Vermont to finish a visit to his mother while I returned to Tucson. I half-wondered whether, after getting him into so wretched a position, all on account of my writing, I'd ever see him again. The communication we'd worked so hard to establish over twenty-five years of marriage was jammed into pure static. Miserable and lonely, I jetted back to Tucson and let myself into the house just in time to snap on that morning's "Oprah Winfrey" show, tape-delayed until 3:30 in Tucson. And it was even worse than it had seemed at the time, a real tour de force of suppressed woman-bashing.

Well, George did come back, of course. And very soon we stopped getting the kind of stares people give you at the credit union or the supermarket when they think you look familiar but aren't sure why, although I'm afraid the receptionists in the dental office still exclaim about our celebrity at every visit. As though getting one's teeth picked at and scoured weren't disagreeable enough.

The candor about my experiences and emotions which caused my *New York Times* letter writer to pity George in the first place has had mixed consequences. These began to become apparent soon after my first book of essays, *Plaintext,* was published. Call me naive if you like, but I was just as pained and surprised by the resistance my work aroused in some people as I was thrilled by the warmth with which others embraced it. I simply hadn't known what to expect. In "On Uttering the Unspeakable," which I wrote originally for a conference called "Literary Women," I try to sort out the significance of these responses. *Remembering the Bone House,* which was only a gleam in my eye at the time of the conference, turned out to be easily as "rude," in the sense defined in the essay, as I'd anticipated. Too rude for its own good, in fact. If I find my thoughts drifting toward ways I could have made it and the work that's followed it politer, and thus more palatable, I make myself reread "On Uttering the Unspeakable." If writers can't take courage from their own work, why should they expect others to?

The need to give myself heart in the face of strong disapproval also precipitated "Faith and Loving in Las Vegas," the only piece in this collection written not to fulfill an assignment but purely to give me the chance to fix and reflect upon an event that moved me profoundly: my first act of civil disobedience. When, after it was published, a reviewer referred to my "liberal pieties," I ground my teeth and writhed. "Pieties" I can live with. A woman who goes to Mass every week leaves herself wide open for such a judgment. "Pieties" is sort of like Brussels sprouts: I don't much like them, but I can get them down. But *"liberal"*? Oh, "liberal" is liver! It gives me the collywobbles. I crave the crunch and bite of radishes.

I want, that is, to grub around underground for the roots connecting experience with belief and action, as "Carnal Acts" begins to do. Lest anyone should think that the assignments a writer takes on (often, but not always, for money) distract her from her "real" work, turning her into a dutiful drudge, "Carnal Acts" speaks otherwise. At the time I wrote it, to read at Colby College, I had nearly finished drafting *Remembering the Bone House,* which had only recently yielded its title; and the ideas I struggled with in the essay illuminated for me the specific nature of the book: not just a memoir, not even a feminist memoir, but a memoir of my life as a female body. Slowly, what I had not permitted myself to speak found voice in the essay and thereafter instructed me in my revision.

This release of radical energy explains why I take assignments, even ones I don't get paid for. True, I'm a good girl, and good girls find it hard to refuse tasks, especially the ones with noble overtones like addressing students or people with disabilities (and often both at once). But I serve myself as well. For one thing, I'm a slow starter, the sort who finds writing so difficult and, yes, terrifying that I'll do anything else that offers itself (remember French phenomenology?) first. Then, too, I'm a relentless self-critic who jettisons most material even before it hits the page. By filling someone else's needs and expectations, I lose track of my own; and through the crack formed by that slight shift of attention, of focus, new ideas bubble and ooze, some of which I'm forced to keep because I *need* them. Otherwise, there I'll be in a Sheraton ballroom in front of a couple of hundred people, spoons poised over their chocolate parfaits, with my mouth hanging open. (I'm not joking about this sort of setting. Once, I was the entertainment at a black-tie fund-raiser, and people said they liked me better than the fashion show the year before.) What a nightmare. I'd even rather write.

Carnal act, then, as carnival act. Praise God for the expectant audience, who calls up out of the writer her own unanticipated joy.

This evocation has been especially valuable to me when I'm asked to address audiences concerned with disability in general, or MS in particular, as on the occasions for the last six essays. I don't want to think about having MS. I don't want to *have* MS to think about. Having to speak of it, aloud, to others, forces me to examine what about life-with-MS (about which I have no choice) is worth having. And celebrating.

In the fall of 1986 I undertook what came to be known in my family as The Great Los Angeles Adventure, which began on a low note when I fell onto a concrete floor on my head and knocked myself out cold. This event taught me, as disagreeable events often will, a number of lessons that I'm glad enough to know but wish I'd been permitted to learn in some other way. It gave me, for instance, a livelier sense than I'd ever had before of the existence of worlds absolutely other than, and perhaps inimical to, the one I occupy and generalize from. During the several hours I lay in the emergency room at the Brotman Medical Center, a black woman with labor pains but without health insurance was bustled into a taxicab and sent away to another hospital. A black security guard who'd tried to stop a robbery had been kicked and pummeled bloody. The robbery had been completed. "You shouldn't ever try to stop them," said the police officer. "They could have guns, and then where would you be?" "I don't know who did it," a black teenager moaned to his mama and another police officer. "I was just getting something out of the trunk of my girlfriend's car when— *blam!*—right in the ass." After consultation, the doctors decided to leave the bullet where it was, and both they and the police released him.

In a sense, my accident forced me briefly into the helpless and violent world these glimpses suggested. The first thing I remember after being wheeled in from the ambulance was a young doctor's earnest face close to mine: "Who did this to you?" "Why—no one," I said. "I did it to myself. I fell." But I, who have seldom been struck and never beaten, understood with a wholly new immediacy that women like me are carried into these places night after night and, whatever they say, they haven't fallen. When George visited me the following weekend, he was drawn into this vision. Eating lunch in an outdoor café on Venice Boulevard, we gradually became aware of the stares—pitying for me, hostile for him—aroused by my battered face. In spite of our innocence, we shrank in humiliation.

On a happier note, I learned that, even in a city of several million strangers (at least if you're white and well dressed and have health insurance), people will take care of you. The doctors and nurses attended me as carefully as their harried lives permitted; and a couple of young physicists from my apartment building who'd been in the group that gathered around me after my fall adopted me, checking on my progress and driving me home from the hospital after my release. Because I travel a good deal, this confidence in strangers makes my life less anxious than it might be. True, I was once verbally abused by a Providence cabby, who told me people like me had no business traveling but ought to stay home where they belonged, but what's one crank among millions of potential caregivers?

These events and lessons were fresh in my memory when I wrote "Challenge: An Exploration," which shares the theme of the essays that follow it: how to live deliberately and responsibly in the face of a chronic incurable degenerative disease that limits physical freedom and satisfaction without turning either to jelly or to stone. It may be possible to carry out this process alone, but I am fortunate in never having had to try. My family has chosen to remain with me, and so when I write about living with MS, inevitably I write about their lives as well. I've thought about revising these essays to broaden their focus, but in the end I've left them as written for a couple of reasons. First, I think they provide a rough but accurate sketch of what can go on in an MS family; and second, I think what goes on in an MS family is universal enough, in style if not in detail, to be recognizable by people unaffected by MS. All groups of people whose lives are bound together are "gifted" in some way, and they share the task of making meaning out of life's ambiguous bounty.

You may feel surprised, even skeptical, at my tendency to concentrate on the positive contributions MS has made to our ways of living in the world and relating to it and one another. To the outside world people like us seldom get the chance to name our blessings, since outsiders assume that chronic illness must offer unmitigated misery and that celebrating as well as bemoaning our lot marks us as either Pollyannas or perverts. Don't be too sure. Once you've tasted George's ricotta-stuffed crêpes with chocolate sauce and Amaretto whipped cream, you may just decide that my increasing incapacity in the kitchen, which has forced him to explore a space from which he had since childhood felt barred, is indeed nothing short of a blessing.

To view your life as blessed does not require you to deny your pain. It simply demands a more complicated vision, one in which a condition or event is not either good or bad but is, rather, both good and bad, not sequentially but simultaneously. In my experience, the more such ambivalences you can hold in your head, the better off you are, intellectually and emotionally. Categorical statements become meaningless. The saddest stories are shot through with humor. You come to tolerate people, ideas, and circumstances wholly at odds with your dreams and desires.

As the luncheon speaker at a conference, I recall, I was seated at a table with the other presenters, among them a psychologist who had recently published a book about MS. He was perhaps ten years younger than I, fair and bearded and balding, with a sweet, almost wistful expression. He appeared only mildly affected by the disease, with a limp caused by characteristic foot drop; he hardly seemed to need his cane. In other words, he looked very much as I had looked for many of the years I'd had MS. I no longer looked that way. Even with my brace and cane, I couldn't totter unassisted more than a few feet, and in public I seldom left my three-wheeled electric scooter. I had no use of my left hand anymore, so my movements were clumsy and lopsided. And I was getting worse. I remembered looking like him, however. I remembered being only slightly crippled. At that time, I tended to avoid gatherings of people with MS, but when I did see people hunched in wheelchairs or scooters, listened to their slurred speech, watched them fumble their coffee cups and forks, my response was clear and adamant: "Oh, no. I can bear the way I am right now, but I could never stand being like that. This far I can go, but no further."

"I was like you once," I said aloud now, turning toward the psychologist, "and I thought then that I couldn't stand being the way I am now." He looked a little startled but politely attentive, torn perhaps between being an MS person and a professional therapist. "And now I am the woman I thought I could never bear to be." Just then the conference leader caught my eye, and I pulled away from the table and got ready to roll up onto the stage and read "I'm Afraid. I'm Afraid. I'm Afraid."

I am still being the woman I thought I could never bear to be. And I am still afraid.

Because I keep as close to the bone of my experience as I can (no matter what I'm writing about, but especially if I'm writing about MS), certain details are apt to emerge over time and, stressed by reiteration, to reveal the concerns currently central to me: just so, in these last few essays, my daughter's presence as a Peace Corps worker in Zaïre, arousing a complicated mix of excitement and alarm and loneliness which flavors my whole life strongly. Also, with the reiteration of such details over time, my work sometimes takes on an inadvertent narrative quality. In "I'm Afraid. I'm Afraid. I'm Afraid.," for example, I was screwing up my courage for a trip to Africa. I wrote "Where I Never Dreamed I'd Go, and What I Did There" shortly after my return; thus, it continues the saga known affectionately in our family as The Amazing Adventures of Anne in Africa.

I wanted to go to Africa as much as I've ever wanted anything, but my physical condition was deteriorating progressively, and I really didn't know whether I could pull it off. In my anxiety I found myself reverting to a kind of infantile prayer that horrifies me when, eavesdropping on my own spirit, I pick up its mumblings: "Please, God, keep me well enough to make this trip. After I get back, I'll be just as sick as you like. I'll even die. But first, please, let me go to Zaïre." I don't even believe in a God who strikes bargains, and certainly not in one who would exact as a price my illness or even my death. Nevertheless, my spirit muttered on, primitive and panicky.

Well, I did get to go, and I'm very glad, too, because since then I've grown even weaker. That's not God's doing. It's just the nature of MS. It makes me wonder, though, whether I've made myself out in these essays to be a pluckier woman than I really am. I'm not keeping my end of that primitive bargain at all well. I'm dragging my feet, and not just metaphorically. As I said to George the other day, "Being in a wheelchair all the time was always something I was going to worry about in the future, and now the future seems to be here." I don't want to enter it, that world of hospital beds, damp sheets, personal attendants, sponge baths, spoon-feeding: all the elements that once made up my nightmares, turning slowly into the furnishings of my days. Debility lies in that direction. And then death. I'll go if I have to, but under protest.

A reviewer once spoke of my "valiant battle against multiple sclerosis." It was a bad review, but I hated this phrase—which I suspect he meant as a compliment—far more than the nastinesses he dispensed. I hated the way he reduced the existence I have painstakingly constructed to the corpses and smoking rubble of a battlefield and set me, a heroic figure, wounded but still defiant, in the middle of the waste: another silly story of the sort little boys make up for their Transformers and GI Joes. Lest you be tempted into a similar maudlin misreading of life with chronic illness, keep this in mind: I am only doing what I have to do. It's enough.

☞ Shape ☜

I am listening to *The Doors' Greatest Hits*. It is Abby's album. She bought it last week, along with something called *Scary Monsters, Super Creeps* by David Bowie, and I was amused that she would spend her carefully hoarded babysitting money on the songs that she heard while she was cutting her teeth and tottering from couch to coffee table to chair and riding on her father's shoulders in peace marches on the commons of all the towns around Boston. But the Doors are popular again, as are the Beatles and Jimi Hendrix and even Cream. These children seem nostalgic for a life they never lived—for *my* life—and I find their nostalgia odd and touching, a kind of statement about the charmed existence I must have had, though I was not much aware of the charm at the time.

Under my fingers a head is taking shape. The afternoon is hot, and the clay against my palms feels as

19

warm as flesh. For several weeks now I have felt heavy, doughy, especially in my head, and my vision has been blurred. But this morning, in spite of the thunderous August heat, I woke to lightness and clarity. That's the part of having multiple sclerosis I find hardest to deal with, the unpredictability with which the symptoms come and go. I just get used to living one way when I shift to another. Today, at last, I felt like working, and I've been at it for a couple of hours now. The head is strange, elongated, with high cheekbones and a pointed chin and protuberant eyes, embryonic somehow, like the head of a six-month fetus in one of those photos by Nilsson. It doesn't look like my usual work at all. I seldom do any part of the human form. I do animals—cats, mostly. There's a good demand for them, and although Michael is generous with what he has, it never seems to be enough, especially now that David is in college. So I can use the money.

Over the music I hear the telephone ring and then stop ringing. Since it's Saturday, the call will be for Abby, and I'm glad I don't have to stop working to answer it. The ringing pushes me back past the Doors, past confused images of newly baked potato bread and "We Shall Overcome" and diapers frozen to the clothesline, of friends drinking burgundy and writing slogans in Magic Marker on white posterboard in the kitchen of the bare white apartment outside Porter Square, back to a much earlier period, when I was just about Abby's age and had fallen in love for the first time. With Allen, a tall skinny boy, red-headed and freckled, who was in love not with me but with World War II battleships and planes. Abby loves me to tell her about Allen, and I charm her sometimes with the story of how I had to battle the battleships and planes, and how every day on the bus ride to and from school I did, though I don't remember now precisely what weapons were in my arsenal, until finally, not long before the prom, I could feel myself coming into focus in Allen's sights. Then began the battle of nerves, as every night I sat at my desk working algebra problems or reading *Romeo and Juliet* while I waited for the telephone, which I pretended not to hear, and for my mother's voice calling, "Pamela, phone for you!"

Allen never did call, but later others did, and I have never quite shaken the slight catch of breath at the ringing of the telephone, which seldom rings anymore for me. Sometimes it does, of course. There are still insurance salesmen and cleaning services for the carpets I don't have and, more important, gallery owners and a few friends, but some of those drifted away when I first got sick, and more when Michael and I got divorced, and the others leave the city every weekend in the summer. For a moment I wish that I still had a lover, that Jeremy would come back, just so I'd have some reason to listen for the telephone. My life, scrubbed of romantic possibilities, is serene, open, but assuredly flat. Come winter I'll get more calls, I think, and then I'll pull out of this funk into which heat and humidity acting on a whimsical nervous system have thrown me. I'll probably even start feeling harassed.

I feel good about the head, which is emerging more and more clearly from the damp brownish clay. One of my friends in the art department at Brandeis has been after me to teach a sculpture course, but I have thought that two trips out there every week would be too tiring.

Looking at the head, I decide to call him on Monday and say that I'll try it for a semester.

Abby comes into my studio and I twist around to look at her. She is wearing a red towel around her body and a purple one around her head. She is a lovely color, almost like my clay, since she's been working every weekday morning this summer as a mother's helper, taking a neighbor's children to a nearby park. She hates the children, who have been raised to treat anyone over four feet tall as a serf, but she likes the money. She is saving for a trip to San Francisco to see her friend Samuel, whose father has just transferred to the zoo there because it has better snakes. Red and purple and brown, she looks sumptuous, like an Aztec princess, and I think, not for the first time, that one of the many gifts Michael gave me was two exotic children, grafted like mangoes onto the apple-stem of my Yankee family.

"Hi, Abby," I say, looking back down at my hands. "Who was on the phone?"

"Harriet. She's back from Nova Scotia." Her voice, raised above the music, sounds high and clear, as though she is shouting from a great distance.

"Did she have a good time?"

"Yeah, so-so, I guess. Can you take us to the movies tonight? We want to see *The Stunt Man*."

"Oh Lord, Abby," I sigh. I want to see *The Stunt Man* too, and she knows it, but I don't want to see it tonight. My left wrist is getting floppy and the small of my back, where the muscles are weakest, feels tight and sore from staying upright for several hours. I want to take a cool bath and make a fruit salad for supper and spend the evening lying in front of the television. "Can't you take the bus?"

"Wouldn't do any good. The movie's rated R."

"Oh damn, of course it is. How about Harriet's father—could he take you?" Harriet's mother died of cancer a couple of years ago, and I feel guilty about suggesting her father. He transports the girls too often as it is. But maybe he wouldn't mind just once more.

"Harriet's father has gone to New York. She's staying with her grandmother, *who doesn't have a license,*" she finishes in a rush, anticipating me.

"I'm sorry, Abby, but not tonight. I've been working very hard this afternoon, and I'm just too tired to go out."

"But we could go to the early show."

"Maybe tomorrow night."

"Je-*sus,* Mother." She snatches at the red towel, which has begun to undrape itself. "No wonder Father left you. He was probably dying of boredom." Her head is down as she tucks the end of the towel between her breasts, but she speaks distinctly. "Harriet's right. You're nothing but a damned cripple."

"Riders on the Storm" ends, and the record clicks off. In the sudden silence I can hear Abby's breath against the back of her right hand; above the palm her eyes are wide. Still clutching the towel with her left hand, she turns and runs out of the studio, kicking the door shut behind her.

The quiet in the room seems creepy. I wipe most of the clay off my hands with a damp rag and then push the swivel chair I work in over to the stereo and turn the record over. My hands have started trembling, as they always do now when I get upset. I have a hard time getting the Doors going again.

What Abby has said seems to me inevitable. I shouldn't feel so shocked. The only real surprise is that it took her so long. After all, we've been living alone together for nearly a year, ever since David left for Emory, longer really, since David's independence kept him out of the house as much as in. But at least he sometimes took Abby with him, skating or sailing or hiking the Appalachian Trail, and she didn't have to depend so much on me for companionship and transportation. At the beginning of the summer, when their father offered to fly them both down to spend their vacation with him, I was relieved that although David accepted, Abby refused, wanting to spend the last bit of time she could with Samuel. I didn't want to face the uncertainty of a summer alone. But maybe she should have gone.

Abby is wrong, of course, about why Michael left me, but I can't think how to tell her that. I don't understand his reasons entirely myself. He never liked explanations. I only know that he began to leave quite a while ago, before he knew there was anything wrong with me, before I was really aware of it myself. His leaving seemed not to have very much at all to do with me personally, in fact. I think that he liked me, that he still likes me. From a distance. Perhaps he was homesick. I don't know. For a while I thought there might be another woman, after a female voice called and asked for "Miguel." But when I told him about the call, he said it was a secretary from the consulate answering a question he had had about his visa, and I suspect that he was telling the truth.

"I'm going home," he told me one afternoon, coming into the studio with a sheaf of the yellow onionskin on which his sister wrote to him, with neat angular black strokes, every week. "My mother is getting worse."

I was still working in wood then, and I had been experimenting with a crude whittled effect, using the big blade of the Swiss army knife David had given me for Christmas. The blade had slipped and bitten into the first knuckle of my left forefinger, and now I was sitting in front of the chunk of pale wood holding an ice cube wrapped in paper towel against the cut. Michael looked at my hands, then went out to the bathroom and came back with scissors, Dermaplast, gauze pads, adhesive tape. He pulled the wet pinkish paper towel away and sprayed the cut.

"Does it hurt?" he asked, wrapping the finger in gauze.

"No, not much."

"I don't think it's too deep." He cut off some strips of tape and wound them loosely around the padded finger.

"Shall I come home with you?" I asked. I knew the answer, but the habit of courtesy between us dictated the question.

"No, I think not," he said. "But thank you for asking." He kissed the finger, as we had always done when patching up Abby or David or each other, and went back out.

Not long afterward I cut myself again, that time on the back of my hand, and I realized that I was getting too clumsy to handle the tools safely, so I gave up wood, though I still think about it, the grain and weight and fragrance.

Once Michael decided to go, he went quickly, quitting his job with the Boston Industrial Mission, settling his affairs with me, and flying out in just over two weeks. I missed him, I still miss him sometimes, but I get as much from his long, meticulous letters as I did from living with him toward the end, maybe more. How can I explain this amiable dissolution of the marriage bond to my passionate fifteen-year-old daughter?

Easier, perhaps, to explain to her about Jeremy, for if anyone was troubled by my being a damned cripple, it was Jeremy, not Michael. I don't think about Jeremy very often anymore, and I'm surprised to be thinking of him again today. Earlier I was remembering how he told me about losing his virginity to a psychology graduate student while "Light My Fire" played over and over on the stereo. He brought the whole clumsy, strained procedure to life in a few sentences, between sips of beer, and I laughed, watching his eyes, his heavy mouth, trying to reconstruct the eighteen-year-old in this aging boy with whom I was falling in love.

I met Jeremy a year ago last spring, not long after Michael left, when he moved to the city and started walking his dog along the river, where I walked my dog, and we had an affair that ended as abruptly as it began. It began with the dogs, of course. Mine was a small mongrel named Thoby Stephen, black with white chest and forepaws and a terrier-style mustache going gray; his was something large and white and purebred which I can still picture clearly but whose name I seem to have forgotten. They found one another on a smoky day in late April in the middle of a plot of red and yellow tulips, in which they snarled and snapped until Jeremy, wading in among the flattened stems and broken petals, hauled Thoby out and shoved him at me, muttering something about keeping my goddamned dog on a leash. His dog was off the leash too, but it seemed egregious to point that out. I snapped Thoby onto the chain; Jeremy leashed his dog; and the two entered a pact of neutrality that permitted Jeremy and me to walk side by side.

Before long we found ourselves hurrying to the river every afternoon, and soon Jeremy asked me to his place for tea, but it turned out that my place was closer, so we went there. Thoby, however, though he'd learned to tolerate Jeremy's dog in a public place, could not bear him on his own territory, and tea turned out to be an awkward affair, punctuated by growls and the baring of teeth. After that, Jeremy and I left the dogs home when we visited each other. We still walked them together frequently, though, and when at the end of the summer I had an attack while Abby and David were camping in the Berkshires, Jeremy came for Thoby twice a day.

But as soon as the children came back, he told me he no longer wanted to sleep with me. That's what he said, sitting on the top step of my front porch pulling a thorn out of one of Thoby's pads with a pair of tweezers: "I no longer want to sleep with you." He dropped the thorn over the railing. Thoby licked Jeremy's cheek once, then settled down to work on the injured paw.

"Why?" I asked, and felt like a fool. I got what I

asked for: Jeremy needed more space in which to be himself, more time to work on his dissertation, more freedom to be with other women if he felt like it. I think he honestly couldn't imagine that a woman could want to live without a man, especially a woman who was likely to be struck helpless at any moment. My man had left me, so I must be looking for another. He looked at my blunt fingers as though they were claws. Perhaps he could actually feel them sink into the flesh of his shoulders. Perhaps he was imagining what it would be like to wake up one morning next to a woman blind, dumb, limbs twitching, bathed in her own urine. I wouldn't blame him. My future is not one to be taken lightly. I was still too weak then to walk Thoby, so when Abby and David went back to school, I gave him to some friends who have an acre of land around their house in Sudbury, and he died not long after. He was an old dog.

When I started going out again, I ran into Jeremy a few times, and he always said something about our still being friends and how we must get together sometime to talk, and I said each time, "Fine. You call me." But he didn't, and after a while I ran into a woman at a watercolor show who knew Jeremy and thought he had moved away, somewhere in the South, Alabama maybe. Since then I've thought of Jeremy off and on, floating through the rank green Alabama countryside in his space like a bubble, his palms and nose pressed to the transparent curve, and I've wondered if he wasn't, in some way, challenging me to break the bubble. If so, he was challenging the wrong person. After twenty years of marriage, I grant space as automatically as the Cambridge Savings Bank pays me five and a quarter on my account. Which is not to say I don't miss Jeremy. I do. And he probably wasn't challenging me anyway. He looked just as happy the last time he walked down the steps, past the day lilies, out into the street, as he ever had.

Some of this I could probably explain to Abby, but I don't want to.

I have been looking at the long blind elegant head in front of me without touching it. The Doors have howled their way through "L.A. Woman" and stopped; the room is once again quiet. I will not do any more work today. Anyway, the head, rough as it is, seems almost finished. I swaddle it in a plastic Rainbo bread bag like an amniotic sac through which it stares blindly at me in the last light of the August afternoon.

Maybe I should take Abby and Harriet to the movies. But I think of throwing together some dinner and putting on my brace and getting into the car and driving to the theater and sitting through the movie and driving home again. I am tired. I am also afraid, I realize. I am afraid of losing Abby. I am afraid that if I refuse to take her to the movies, she will leave me. She will decide to go live with her father, and then I will be alone. Michael has gone, and David, and Thoby, and Jeremy, and if Abby goes there will be no one in the house but me and the spooky striped cat Abby brought me from the Humane Society after I had to give Thoby away. I will become a cartoon character—Old Woman with Pussycat—something straight out of George Booth. I don't even know if I can keep the silly beast in fresh food and kitty litter.

I am afraid, and the room is getting dark. I can

hardly see through the dusk. I have been picking the clay from under my fingernails, but my hands still feel puckered and gritty. If I take Abby and Harriet to the movies, then tomorrow I may be too tired to work. I have been thinking about hands, a torso, Michael's high tight buttocks the first time I ever saw them, pale as stone in the half-light of a rainy late-winter afternoon.

I fish my cane from under the chair and get up. I'm still shaky. I grope my way to David's old room, which Abby has taken over, with one hand against the wall, feeling like a cripple. The door is open. In some indefinable way, the room seems feminine, in spite of David's old "Star Trek" bedspreads and his Sierra Club posters all over the walls. Maybe it's just Abby herself, cross-legged on the bed nearest the window. She has shed the towels and is wearing cutoffs and my old Bruce Springsteen T-shirt. Her dark hair, parted in the middle, falls straight and damp almost to her waist. Crying has lengthened and thinned her face. Her eyes seem too large. If she goes to her father, I will be very lonely.

"Abby," I say, "come." I take her hand, and it lies against my palm as limp and hot as it used to when I walked her to and from nursery school. "Come and see the funny head I've just done."

❧ "Hers" Columns ❧

Disability. July 9, 1987.

For months now I've been consciously searching for representations of myself in the media, especially television. I know I'd recognize this self because of certain distinctive, though not unique, features: I am a forty-three-year-old woman crippled by multiple sclerosis; although I can still totter short distances with the aid of a brace and a cane, more and more of the time I ride in a wheelchair. Because of these appliances and my peculiar gait, I'm easy to spot even in a crowd. So when I tell you I haven't noticed any woman like me on television, you can believe me.

    Actually, last summer I did see a woman with multiple sclerosis portrayed on one of those medical dramas that offer an illness-of-the-week like the daily special at your local diner. In fact, that was the whole point of the show: that this poor young woman had MS.

She was terribly upset (understandably, I assure you) by the diagnosis, and her response was to plan a trip to Kenya while she was still physically capable of making it, against the advice of the young, fit, handsome doctor who had fallen in love with her. And she almost did make it. At least, she got as far as a taxi to the airport, hotly pursued by the doctor. But at the last she succumbed to his blandishments and fled the taxi into his manly protective embrace. No escape to Kenya for this cripple.

Capitulation into the arms of a man who uses his medical powers to strip one of even the urge toward independence is hardly the sort of representation I had in mind. But even if the situation had been sensitively handled, according the woman her right to her own adventures, it wouldn't have been what I'm looking for. Such a television show, as well as films like *Duet for One* and *Children of a Lesser God*, in taking disability as its major premise, excludes the complexities that round out a character and make her whole. It's not about a woman who happens to be physically disabled; it's about physical disability as the determining factor of a woman's existence.

Take it from me, physical disability looms pretty large in one's life. But it doesn't devour one wholly. I'm not, for instance, Ms. MS, a walking, talking embodiment of a chronic incurable degenerative disease. In most ways I'm just like every other woman of my age, nationality, and socioeconomic background. I menstruate, so I have to buy tampons. I worry about smoker's breath, so I buy mouthwash. I smear my wrinkling skin with lotions. I put bleach in the washer so my family's undies won't be dingy. I drive a car, talk on the telephone, get runs in my

32

pantyhose, eat pizza. In most ways, that is, I'm the advertisers' dream: Ms. Great American Consumer. And yet the advertisers, who determine nowadays who will get represented publicly and who will not, deny the existence of me and my kind absolutely.

I once asked a local advertiser why he didn't include disabled people in his spots. His response seemed direct enough: "We don't want to give people the idea that our product is just for the handicapped." But tell me truly now: If you saw me pouring out puppy biscuits, would you think these kibbles were only for the puppies of cripples? If you saw my blind niece ordering a Coke, would you switch to Pepsi lest you be struck sightless? No, I think the advertiser's excuse masked a deeper and more anxious rationale: To depict disabled people in the ordinary activities of daily life is to admit that there is something ordinary about disability itself, that it may enter anybody's life. If it is effaced completely, or at least isolated as a separate "problem," so that it remains at a safe distance from other human issues, then the viewer won't feel threatened by her or his own physical vulnerability.

This kind of effacement or isolation has painful, even dangerous consequences, however. For the disabled person, these include self-degradation and a subtle kind of self-alienation not unlike that experienced by other minorities. Socialized human beings love to conform, to study others and then to mold themselves to the contours of those whose images, for good reasons or bad, they come to love. Imagine a life in which feasible others—others you can hope to be like—don't exist. At the least you might conclude that there is something queer about you, something ugly or foolish or shameful. In the extreme, you might feel as though you don't exist, in any meaningful social sense, at all. Everyone else is "there," sucking breath mints and splashing on cologne and swigging wine coolers. You're "not there." And if not there, nowhere.

But this denial of disability imperils even you who are able-bodied, and not just by shrinking your insight into the physically and emotionally complex world you live in. Some disabled people call you TAPs, or Temporarily Abled Persons. The fact is that ours is the only minority you can join involuntarily, without warning, at any time. And if you live long enough, as you're increasingly likely to do, you may well join it. The transition will probably be difficult from a physical point of view no matter what. But it will be a good bit easier psychologically if you are accustomed to seeing disability as a normal characteristic, one that complicates but does not ruin human existence. Achieving this integration, for disabled and able-bodied people alike, requires that we insert disability daily into our field of vision: quietly, naturally, in the small and common scenes of our ordinary lives.

Illiteracy. July 16, 1987.

Week after week Henrietta comes to clean my house. Despite her good humor, I don't think she much likes this kind of work, but it's all she can get without a high-school diploma. She is a small, plain, soft-spoken woman of thirty-three, the divorced mother of four children, ages five to thirteen. She knows where their father is, but they never see him and he contributes nothing to their support. The five of them survive on payments from Aid to Families with Dependent Children of $4,236 a year plus what I give her each week.

I met Henrietta through my husband, who teaches in an adult-education program, helping people to earn a general equivalency diploma. Without such certification, they are disqualified from all but the most menial and irregular work. His students are predominantly women—most of them mothers, many in middle age—placed in the program by the Arizona Department of Economic Security as part of an effort to shift them from public assistance to full employment. For their attendance they receive three dollars a day. Funds and staff keep dwindling as the federal administration, despite recent protestations of concern about adult illiteracy, continues to slash at the program's resources. But the women keep coming.

Not long ago illiteracy had its promised fifteen minutes of fame, which gave an emotional (though not a financial) boost to programs like the one my husband teaches in. During that time I was surprised that women's groups didn't take up the issue eagerly, for certain basic facts about women's lives make the question of illiteracy a particularly lively one for them. Take, for instance, the now familiar results of a 1985 study of divorced families by Lenore J. Weitzman, a sociologist: In the year following the divorce, the average husband's standard of living rises 42 percent while that of the wife and children falls 73 percent. Too, in the past decade, teenage pregnancies among all ethnic groups have increased sharply, and many of these very young women are choosing to try to raise their babies on their own. Some researchers predict that, by the year 2000, virtually all the people living below the poverty line in this country will be women and children.

The problems that underlie such statistics are extraordinarily complex, and I don't mean to imply that we can sweep them away simply by teaching women to read, write, and handle fractions. But neither do I belittle such capabilities. The woman solely responsible for herself and her children occupies a marginal position, socially and economically, at best. If she's illiterate, she may be pushed outside society's margins altogether.

The illiterate woman is essentially helpless to shape her own life. Unable to find work at wages that will support her family, she must live on public assistance, which is inadequate for her needs and which, more importantly, reinforces her passivity. In such a situation, earning a GED can be of enormous practical significance. Not only can she now qualify for numerous jobs previously closed to her, but she becomes eligible for further training that may prepare her to work outside traditionally female occupations, which traditionally offer both low pay and low status. Moreover, she can assume an active stance, earning rather than receiving the money with which she feeds and shelters herself and her family. Thus, her entire relationship to society is transformed.

If, as seems to be the case, the majority of our children are going to be raised by single mothers, then the impact of a woman's literacy extends beyond her own social position and self-esteem. The children of a literate mother benefit enormously, of course, from the bedtime storytelling, the little notes, the help with a subtraction problem, the trips to the library—all the small commonplaces of literate life. Even more important, they see their mother, perhaps their only role model in the home, as a competent, self-defined, and active element in their lives. Literacy may not be genetically inheritable, but it is passed down from generation to generation nonetheless.

Women are succeeding in these ways. Take my husband's student Rita, for example. The child of migrant workers, she loved school but could never keep up, so at fourteen she dropped out and married. She has had nine "blessings," as she calls them; when the youngest started school, she went back herself and earned her general equivalency diploma. In fact, she was the student speaker at her graduation. She now works in a program for needy senior citizens and attends our local community college. Given the chance for such accomplishment, most women will take it. And though they're often timid at first, with encouragement most of them thrive.

Writing an article about women's illiteracy seems futile on the face of it. After all, my audience can, by definition, read; they don't need to be persuaded of the virtues of literacy. But they may not have reflected on the ways in which literate women can work to swell their own ranks. They can, for one thing, volunteer in programs like my husband's, enabling an overtaxed staff with limited resources to reach further and more deeply. They can also lobby for an increase in those resources. The women entering these programs need ample support in the form of stipends, book allowances, day-care services, flexible class hours, social and vocational counseling, and the like. These would cost significantly less than a fleet of B-1 bombers, maybe even less than one B-1 bomber, and they would provide a more solid line of defense. Because at bottom, the strongest country is not the one with the classiest weapons and most complicated technology. The strongest country is the one whose citizens, certain of their skills and worth, believe that they can take care of themselves and one another.

Commencement. July 23, 1987.

My daughter has always been slight, compact, but she plants her feet firmly, heels first, as she walks. She has little hands and a small, slightly pointed face framed just now by a tumble of reddish curls. In her slim-waisted white cotton dress, trimmed with lace on the wide collar and flounced skirt, and her black ankle boots, she might be graduating in her great-great-grandmother's class of 1901. She has shrugged her heavy black gown over her dress and set her mortarboard square on her curls, and she strides by us looking solemn and steamy. She doesn't know where we are sitting, and when we speak her name she turns with a start, her mouth an oval of surprise captured forever by Polaroid.

The weather and the campus provide a flawless setting. Despite a freak late-April snowstorm not three weeks before, the vegetation is burgeoning: dogwood, lilac, rhododendron, azalea stain the atmosphere with colors and scents that stun my senses, tuned now to Arizona's more muted spring. Far from needing the light woolen jacket I brought to thaw my desert-thinned blood, I'm grateful for the spotty shade of a nearby tree. Limp with light and warmth, I watch the women—687 of them—file to their seats and the sheriff of Hampshire County, his face wet and ruddy beneath his top hat, declare these proceedings open.

My own graduation, though it took place on a campus just as picturesque, I don't remember as half so lovely. My dress wasn't quite right, for one thing. (This is the surviving memory of most of the significant events of my life: that my dress wasn't quite right.) Our dresses were supposed to be white, but mine, made for me by my mother for some other occasion, was embroidered with tiny yellow flowers. The day was overcast and damp, and my spirits were equally gray. College had seemed one long survival test, which I had passed, but without distinction. Although surrounded by proud and loving family, I was lonely for the one person who made my survival seem worthwhile, my husband, sailing in large aimless circles on a radar picket ship in the North Atlantic.

I would go on immediately, I knew, to travel to New Mexico for a friend's wedding, and in the fall to teach school, and eventually to have children. But these ventures all required leaps into unknown territory—the desert, the classroom, the nursery—and I was afraid that they too would turn out aimless and undistinguished. These feelings are symptomatic of depression, I know now, and if I'd been properly medicated I might have been free of them. But I don't think they're unusual, even for people who aren't clinically depressed, at such radical junctures as leaving college, entering marriage, changing jobs, leaving one house for another. The comfortingly familiar past slides away and leaves one gasping at the vertiginous brink of what can seem, to the inexperienced, a void. But in reality it is only the leading edge of what will become, and surprisingly soon, the comfortingly familiar past.

Now, twenty-three years later, I am watching my daughter's commencement exercises from my wheelchair. My multiple sclerosis has gotten much worse in recent months, and I'm safe only if I stay put; a couple of days ago, trying to walk and read a letter at the same time, I fell flat on my face and shattered the edges of three front teeth, which are now painted on temporarily in plastic. Beside me, holding my hand, my husband (the same one) is recovering from the removal of a second melanoma. A few months ago his father died, reminding us that nothing now stands between ourselves and death; and we are trying to help his mother settle into her grief as well as into her new apartment, furnishing it to her own tastes and needs.

At this sweet moment, waiting to hear my daughter's name announced, I am suddenly, perfectly happy, in a way I couldn't have dreamed at my own graduation. If anyone had told me then that by the time I was forty-three I would be crippled and George would have cancer and my beloved family would have begun to die, I would have cried out (I did a lot of crying out in those days), "Oh no! I could never survive such pain!" But if anyone had told me that, in the presence of these realities, I would find myself, without warning, pierced by joy, I would have been stunned speechless, certain that my informant was either perverse or outright mad.

I wish that I could jump up (a move that, in reality, would probably result in the loss of the rest of my teeth) and hug my daughter and all her classmates in a gargantuan embrace and shout to them, "Listen! No matter how happy you think you are today, you will be happier, I promise you. You can't imagine the women you will grow into, how large those women's spirits will become, stretching and stretching to encompass the challenges their lives will proffer. Take all these challenges as gifts, no matter how dubious their value seems at the time. They'll come in handy one day, you'll see. They'll open you up for joy."

But if I started jumping and hugging and shouting, the director of security, who happens to be hovering several feet to my right (why here? what does he know?), would doubtless lug me bodily to the ambulance parked just outside the archway back there, and my daughter would be mortified at having my perversity and madness go public. Better I should bow my head politely for the benediction and whisper my message to myself. My own life promises to grow more complicated and difficult still, and I will need my own words of encouragement: You don't yet know the woman you will become, Nancy; you will be happier, in ways wholly new to you, than you now dream.

"God save the Commonwealth of Massachusetts!" shouts the sheriff, and the pipers stomp and skirl at the head of the recession. This time Anne knows where we are, and she lights her sunny smile straight at the lens. We give this proper composition to her grandmother, whose camera we've been using, and keep the round-mouthed one for ourselves: Anne entering her future in the only way any of us can, unfocused and surprised.

Home. July 30, 1987.

My husband is forever running away from home. Though the pattern is familiar to me, I never consciously recognized it until, a couple of months ago, my daughter and I borrowed his car for a trip to a nearby town. We were gone perhaps four hours, during which, George told us, he had gone to a local park to sit under a tree reading a book and listening to Bach on my little tape player. Lacking his accustomed means of escape, he'd borrowed Anne's bicycle, its twenty-four-inch wheels barely large enough for her compact frame, and, knees knocking chin, pumped the mile or so to the park and back. We have grass and trees at our house, and books, and a fair-sized stereo with several Bach recordings; so his jaunt can't have fulfilled any practical lack. "Oh Lord," I suddenly realized, "he can't bear to stay here even a few hours. He's driven to get away."

I have long known that George and I live in different worlds. (He doesn't know this, for which reason he believes me crazy, as, according to the terms of his world, I may well be.) But for most of our twenty-four years of marriage, I believed that these worlds were, or at least ought to be, roughly similar, and deviances between them saddened and frightened and shamed me grievously, signs of some mysterious mutual infidelity. I have come to terms slowly over the last few years, however, with the radical nature of their disjunctures. Nowhere have such disparities thrust themselves at me more sharply than in the ways in which he and I relate to the structure that shelters us: "house," "home."

Because George doesn't much talk about this relationship, I'm not certain how he perceives it. But persistently I find myself calling to mind one of James Thurber's most famous cartoons, entitled "Home." In it a tiny man quails before a looming Victorian house whose roofline has dissolved, with Thurberesque ambiguity, into the profile of an enormous glowering woman, poised to gulp him down whole. George is of ordinary size, and our house of modest proportions. But I wonder if he—and perhaps other men raised by mothers who "made homes" where they waited after school each day to ply their boys with milk and chocolate-chip cookies and famished questions about their daily accomplishments out there in the world—doesn't quake a little before plunging across the screened porch into the lighted maw that awaits him. If he, like Thurber, sees "home" as a spiritual deathtrap, even if only at the subliminal level, no wonder he flees it whenever he decently can.

How different are my responses to the house from his. I love being there. I leave it reluctantly and return to it gladly. Sometimes I wander through it celebrating its delights: the day lilies in the whiskey barrel on the front porch; the tin cross above the rough-hewn mantel; the little cobalt tiles in the kitchen; the funny bathroom, all archways and alcoves. Sometimes I plot improvements: bathroom wallpaper with giant rose-colored phoenixes, say, or a ceiling fan in the stuffy guest room. I identify with it so intensely that when George ignores a torn screen, I feel neglected; when he runs away to the park, I am abandoned.

The closest we have ever come to divorce was a couple of years ago when we failed to agree about heating our house. George enjoys feeling cold, a sensation a little hard to come by in the desert, and so when he gets up, well before me, he leaves the thermostat turned down. I don't mind, nestled under the quilt with our cat Vanessa Bell snug against my hip, but as soon as I get up, I chill quickly. At that time, I had asked him repeatedly to turn up the thermostat before I got up. He'd said he would. He didn't. Morning after morning I hunched over my juice and cereal shuddering while the aged furnace labored to warm the air in the leaky old converted Chinese grocery where we lived.

Life on the whole didn't seem to be going well at that time. George left the house before seven in the morning to work at the Casa María Soup Kitchen before going to school. He taught in both morning and evening programs, returning not long before I was ready for bed. Weekends were eaten up by racquetball games and hunger marches and retreats and meetings of Catholics for Peace and Justice. Since each activity was physically or spiritually worthier than the last, I was ashamed to complain, but I was lonely and unhappy. So I sought the counsel of a nun I knew who could understand the nature of my dilemma. And what I found myself blurting out to her was that I was freezing to death in my own house. At that moment in Sister Ursula's sun-warmed office I suddenly understood the metaphorical significance of "my house" for me: my self, of course, but more: my marriage.

"Tell George to turn up the heat," Sister Ursula advised. So I made a date with him for lunch, and on a sun-drenched terrace, right over the chips and salsa, I told him he was chilling me to the bone.

"Yes," he said, "I guess I've pretty well given up on us." Men seem given to such unilateral decision making in a society that hypes individualism the way ours does.

"Well, you might have checked with me first. Because I haven't. And whenever there's an 'us,' it takes two to give up on it."

And so he's stayed, at least for now. I wish I could end this little tale "and they lived happily ever after," because in fact we have been pretty happy since then. We've moved to another house, less leaky, and George turns the thermostat up before I begin to shiver. But on occasion he still runs away from home, for whatever private reasons drive him. And I still sometimes perceive this pattern as rejection, abandonment. Marriages, like houses, haven't got "ever afters." The stucco chips off and the cat falls through the screen and the bathroom drain runs slow. If you don't want the house falling down around your ears, you just plain have to learn to wield a trowel and a hammer and a plunger. And all that activity helps to keep you warm.

Fungi. August 6, 1987.

Auntie E crosses the damp lawn waving a branch at me. "Have you ever seen one of these?" she asks, thrusting out a bit of cedar with something bright wobbling near the end.

I recoil. I have never seen anything more immediately repulsive. Even Sigourney Weaver's heart would lurch. At least the aliens she faced were fabricated by human intelligence and thus, at some level of nightmare, recognizable, even comprehensible. The film viewers peering through trembling fingers *knew* them. Nothing remotely human cooked this creation up. It is absolutely alien.

After a moment stiff with shock, I see it is a fungus. This soggy wooded hillside in Vermont provides ideal media for fungi, and for a while when I was visiting regularly I took a desultory amateur interest in mycology. Here is the only place I ever found a fetid russula, and a fly amanita, not the deadliest of these lovely mushrooms, as well. But I've never seen a specimen of this sort, a cocoa-colored sphere attached to the cedar twig, out of which spring tapered tentacles of muddy orange. Under my fingers these bounce and quiver like those rubbery insects, Kreepy-Krawlies I think they're called, children delight in squandering their money on in amusement-park gift shops. The fungus isn't actually unpleasant to the touch: dry and cool and resilient.

Auntie E isn't sure what it's called, but later a local resident tells us that it's apple-cedar rust, which shuttles between apple and cedar trees in its life cycle. Its cedar host remains unharmed, but infected apple trees die, their bark blackened and curling away from the trunks. Auntie E, her husband, and my daughter tramp over to a stand of cedars maybe a hundred feet from the house and find some as big as a baby's head. From where I sit I can clearly see, now that I'm looking for them, orange smudges staining the shadowy branches.

I am still appalled by the sight of one up close, but I am wonderstruck as well. The world, I think again as I do more and more often in my advancing age, contains more marvels than I will ever meet or understand. And hideous though I think this one is, from the apple-cedar rust's point of view it is simply being its own part of the astonishingly intricate patterns of creation, as I am while I scrutinize it. ("But Mom," says my daughter with the new degree in biochemistry, "the apple-cedar rust hasn't got a point of view." And in fact, unbeknownst to her, I know that. But as part of the discipline of removing myself from the center of the universe, I find it useful to assign even fungi a point of view and then try to occupy a fungicentric universe.) Apple-cedar rust is as it must be.

Three weeks before this botanical discovery, my husband had a second melanoma removed. The first was a mole, and the doctors felt 95 percent certain that they'd "got it all." But a year and a half later it reappeared, this time in a lymph node under his right arm. For the couple of days between its discovery and the surgery, we could hope that it was something else, but as soon as the surgeon saw the node, bigger than a marble and black, he knew. He came and explained the situation to me, and later to George, as frankly as we could hope for, and so did the oncologist he referred us to. But all they could tell us, really, was that we'll all have to wait and see what happens next.

While George was struggling to emerge from the

47

anesthesia sufficiently so that I could take him home, I sat by the high bed and watched his face. The surgery wasn't extensive, and his color was good, though his eyes looked bruised. But he seemed immeasurably removed from me, beyond my touch, beyond my rescue. And I knew suddenly that I was seeing what my future might well be, a future of bedside vigils during which George wanders further and further until he goes for good. Somewhere in his drowsy flesh, solid and chill under my clinging fingers, another cancerous cell might lurk, and another, waiting to lodge in lung or bone or brain, there to multiply into alien black beings the surgeon one day may not be able to carve out and discard.

For the truth is that this multifarious world that holds George and me and apple-cedar rust also holds melanoma. And from the melanoma's point of view (which I know it doesn't have), it is not a hideous aberration in the righteous scheme of things, to be knifed and poisoned and eradicated, leaving the world a better, purer place. It is itself part of the scheme of things, an intricate and ingenious process for self-replication and thus survival. It belongs.

I don't know why. And I wish it didn't. *My* world would be—well, perhaps not better and purer—but certainly an easier place without it. A few months ago I read Susan Kenney's novel *In Another Country* and thrilled at the depth of courage her central character develops as she survives her husband's slow dying of cancer. Then, not long ago, a friend called me intrepid. But I'm only as brave as I have to be, I reminded her. And I do not want to have to be this brave.

All the same, I'll do, like any woman, what has to be done. I'm glad of the reminder, though, from an agglomeration of cells elaborately organized into a brown globe with wriggly orange tentacles, that no evil genius is out to get George or me or the innocent blasted apple trees, no alien invader blighting an Edenic dream. Nothing stands "outside." Everything belongs. We're all weaving some cosmic tapestry of which I've been able to glimpse only a few threads. If it has a design, I'll never know it, nor will the others. We're all just here, for now, each doing what has to be done.

Politeness. August 13, 1987.

In her stunning memoir of bicultural girlhood, *The Woman Warrior*, Maxine Hong Kingston writes, "There is a Chinese word for the female *I*—which is 'slave.' Break the women with their own tongues!" English contains no such dramatic instance of the ways in which language shapes women's reality. We can, after all, use the same "I" as men do. We can, but we're not supposed to, at least not often. In myriad ways the rules of polite discourse in this country serve, among other purposes, not to enslave but certainly to silence women and thus to prevent them from uttering the truth about their lives.

     Seldom are such rules spoken out loud. Indeed, part of their force arises from their implicitness, which makes them seem natural and essential. They vary in detail, I think, from generation to generation, region to region, class to class, though they stifle communication in similar ways. Here, roughly put, are a few of the ones I've learned to obey in the company of men. (The issues of polite discourse among women deserve a study of their own.) If, in a fit of wishful thinking, you're inclined to dismiss them as passé, spend a few hours in the classrooms and corridors of a coeducational high school or college. We haven't actually come all that far, baby.

Rule 1: Keep quiet. If at all possible, a woman should remain perfectly mute. She should, however, communicate agreement with the men around her eloquently through gestures and demeanor. Think, for instance, of the presidents' wives. The first First Lady I remember was Mamie Eisenhower, and from then on my head holds a gallery of film clips and still photos of women in the proper polite posture: Jackie and Lady Bird and Pat and Betty and Rosalynn and above all Nancy, eyes widened and glittering, polished lips slightly parted in breathless wonder, heads tilted to gaze upward at the sides of their husband's faces. Not one yawns or rolls her eyes (much less speaks unless spoken to). Now, if I were elected president, my husband (who dotes on me, by the way) would fall asleep during my inaugural address. There he'd be in the photos, eyes closed, mouth sagging, head rolled to one side, maybe a bit of spittle trickling into his beard. He wouldn't mean to be rude. He's just inclined toward narcolepsy.

Even if you're tempted to break this rule of silence, some man will probably jump in and rescue you from yourself. As Carol Tavris and Carole Wade note in their text on sex differences, *The Longest War*, in mixed conversations men interrupt more freely, and speak at greater

length, than women. So you won't get too much chance
to be rude.

*Rule 2: If you must talk at all, talk about something he's
interested in.* If your feelings are hurt by stifled yawns and
retreating backs, dig out this old chestnut. It's still in
force. Try not to think of all the women who've used up
brain cells memorizing the batting averages of every out-
fielder in Red Sox history or the difference between the
Apollonian and the Dionysian in Nietzsche, depending
on their intended target, instead of reflecting on the
spiritual dilemma of women denied vocations to the
priesthood by the Catholic Church or the effect on human
reproductive systems of even a "limited" nuclear war or
the like.

*Rule 3: If you must mention your own concerns, deprecate
them prettily.* The greatest rudeness in a woman is to appear
to take herself seriously. My husband's indictment of
feminism, for example, and he's not alone in it, is that
feminists "lack a sense of humor." As members of Catholics for Peace and Justice, we both support Sanctuary and
Witness for Peace activities; and in our pained discussions
of human rights issues in Central America I have never
heard him criticize Salvadoran and Guatemalan refugees
or Sandinista peasants for lacking a sense of humor about
their disappeared relatives, their burned infirmaries and
bombed buses, their starvation and terror. Nor should he.
But no more should he expect women to crack jokes when
they are enraged by the malnutrition, rapes, and batter-
ings of their sisters and the system that makes such occur-
rences inevitable.

Actually, in the right places most of the women I

know laugh heartily (even though a belly laugh isn't as polite as a giggle). But they weep in the right places too. "Lighten up," men tell women who grow passionate about the conditions of their lives. "What *is* all this whining?" one wrote to me last week in a "fan letter." When we are the subjects of our speaking, our voices are too "shrill," "strident"; our tongues are too "sharp"; we are "shrews," "Xanthippes," "termagants," "fishwives." All these words have in common the denigration of women's speech. By ridiculing or trivializing women's utterance, men seek to control what is and is not considered important, weighty, worthwhile in the world.

I, for one, was an awfully well-bred girl who grew into a Yankee lady. From infancy, the language slipped into my mouth was scrubbed as clean as my rattles and teething rings; and to this day, I wince at the possibility I might be thought rude. A man's sneer shrivels me. But I guess that's just what I'm going to have to be: rude. Because if women are ever going to be really heard, people (including women themselves) are going to have to get used to the sound of their voices and to the subjects they believe worth discussing. So I, for one, intend to keep telling the truth about my life as a woman: what I see, who I love, where I hurt, why I laugh.

And you? Tell me, out loud, who are you?

ᘒ On Uttering the Unspeakable ᘒ

When my son Matthew was three or so, he hurtled into our living room one day, blubbering: "M-M-Michael hit me."

"Why," I asked, "did Michael hit you?" Michael was a largish boy, maybe eight, and I was inclined to run right out and give him an earful about picking on someone his own size, but I thought I'd best get my facts straight.

"Because I said 'b-b-bullshit' to him."

"Oh," I said. "Well." I tried to sort through the ethics of it. "I don't think people should hit other people, ever. But a word like 'bullshit' can make someone angry, and sometimes angry people do hit."

"What's wrong with it?" piped up Anne, who'd followed her brother through the door. "Marlisa says it all the time."

"Do you guys know what bullshit is?" I asked. They shook their heads. "It's BM," I explained, relying on a family euphemism, "that comes from bulls." They nodded solemnly.

"Now, you can use any words you want to me," I went on. "But Grandma is coming to visit in a couple of weeks, and if you say 'bullshit' to her she'll fall to the floor in a faint and we'll have to pick her up and take care of her. So don't." They didn't—not to Grandma, not to anyone else for a good long time.

Years after these first instructions to my children about polite discourse, just as my book of essays *Plaintext* was published, a friend of my mother's came from the East to Arizona to visit her. She read my book during her stay but, Mother allowed afterward, she didn't think much of it because many of the matters I discussed in it "just weren't very nice": that I was raped by a man I had once loved; that I've had trouble mothering my children; that the power relationships implicit in sexual acts frighten me; that I have more than once tried to kill myself. And suddenly I understood: *Plaintext* had said some intellectual equivalent of "bullshit" to Mother's Yankee houseguest. In its own way, the book violates the rules of polite discourse and marks *me* as "not very nice." Ann Rosalind Jones notes of women writing in the Renaissance, "The link between loose language and loose living arises from a basic association of women's bodies with their speech: a woman's accessibility to the social world beyond the household through speech was seen as intimately connected to the scandalous openness of her body"—and that connection continues today. For a number of people, even those considerably younger than Mother's houseguest, my writing appears to function as the verbal equivalent of sprawling with my legs spread or exposing my bosom (if only I had such a thing) in a tight, low-cut black sweater.

As Mother would want you to understand, I was brought up to know better. As the eldest child in a well-educated middle-class family living on the North Shore of Massachusetts in the 1950s, I endured at least as much regulation of my language as of my dress and behavior. Some quite ordinary words, "stinker," for example, were off limits in my household, so that when an adored teacher once muttered "Shut up!" at me in unteacherly but well-earned irritation, I had an attack of hysterics— wholly baffling to him, I'm sure—more appropriate to having been told to go fuck myself in the ear. Actually, he'd have been better off saying that, since at thirteen I don't think I'd ever heard "fuck," much less knew what it meant.

This last statement reflects the fact that, in the discourse of my youth, not only certain words but, more important, certain subjects were forbidden. My grandfather was an alcoholic, but I was nearly grown before I glimpsed the fact that his ten-day "business trips" were actually binges and that's why my grandmother grieved and the whole family grumbled while he was away; I thought anger was just what you felt whenever a man went away and left you behind. Just before having a stroke, a family friend had gotten a girl pregnant and so "had" to marry her, slurring his vows to her one word at a time in front of their sad parents and the family minister. From the solemnity and whispers and shaken heads I could tell there was something shameful about this whole business; but I thought the shame had to do with sickness.

Later, I was forced to participate in this conspiracy of silence myself. When I was ten, my mother told me some of the facts of life and enjoined me to say nothing of them to my sister, two years younger; Mother would impart them herself to Sally when her time came. The following year, Mother remarried, still young enough for there to be talk of a second family. One day, as we swayed high in the branches of a catalpa tree in front of our aunt's house, Sally turned to me and said, "I asked Mummy when she was going to have a baby, and she said you have to make certain preparations first. What did she mean?" I had some imprecise and academic notion, gleaned from a book Mother had given me called *The Stork Didn't Bring You,* but of course I'd been sworn to secrecy and couldn't communicate it to Sally (which, for the sake of accuracy in her sex education, may have been just as well). "I can't tell you," I stammered. Sally scrambled down the tree and took off for home in tears of fury. I clung to a branch, lonely for my sister, as though I knew already that we would never be perfectly open with one another again. And at some point—perhaps even then—I determined that I wanted no knowledge I couldn't share with all the world.

After my marriage at nineteen, I learned that there were universes of discourse so constricted as to make my family look positively ribald in its openness. When I went into labor with Matthew, for instance, George and I drove

Anne through the April dawn to stay with his parents.

"We're off to the hospital now," I told his mother with determined cheer.

"Are you sick?" Mum asked.

"No, I'm not sick," I said, thinking this woman must have had a sudden amnesiac attack. How could she have forgotten this bulge I'd been lugging in front of me for over eight months? "I'm in labor."

"Oh," she almost whispered. "That's what I meant."

In that family, I gradually learned, one never utters anything even faintly disagreeable, and huge chunks of human experience are at least faintly disagreeable. One winter I had to break the news to Mum and Dad that my little sister was getting a divorce. Clearly, a unit themselves for over fifty years, they disapproved.

"The key to a happy marriage, I always say," said Dad, "is being able to keep your mouth shut." Mum, tucked close beside him on the couch, kept her mouth shut.

Less than a year after this exchange, that marriage, genuinely happy whatever its terms, came to an end with Dad's death, and Mum spent the following few months with us while she acclimated herself to widowhood. During that time she misplaced a little copper pillbox, souvenir of one of their trips together, and grieved for it for weeks.

"When the cleaning woman found it in a cup on the sideboard," I said, recounting the incident to Dad's sister, "Mum was wonderfully happy. I think it acted as a symbol of their life together, and getting it back made

Dad seem a little less dead to her."

"Oh," his sister shuddered, "don't write that. Please, don't ever write that!"

I suspect that what I might have written would violate no discursive rule. I think she was grasping the occasion to insinuate a larger message: not "don't write *that*" but "don't write *at all.*" A tongue like mine, given to revealing the small, intimate details of family life, ought to be silenced utterly.

But surely, you may be thinking as I poke among these muffled memories, there's nothing wrong with a little politeness, is there? Well, no, of course not, if what you mean by politeness is saying, for instance, "Would you please pass me the salt?" instead of "Pass the salt, will yuh?" I'm obviously not talking about salt, however, but about the realities of women's lives, which get distorted or even effaced by permitted language: Childbirth may become sickness. Intercourse may vanish altogether. I focus on women's lives here not just because a woman's life is the one I live but because, according to the French feminist theory that has shaped my thinking, discursive constraints function most stringently to repress the feminine in human experience.

In her essay, "Professions for Women," Virginia Woolf describes the woman writer brought up short in her creative reverie by the thought of "something, something about the body, about the passions, which it was unfitting for her as a woman to say. Men, her reason told her, would be shocked. The consciousness of what men will say of a woman who speaks the truth about her passions had roused her. . . .

"Women writers," she goes on, ". . . are impeded by the extreme conventionality of the other sex." Woolf understands who the gatekeepers of language and literature have always been: men tell women (sometimes even each other) when to keep their mouths shut; men deny permission to speak in certain ways about particular experiences.

In the past, this denial was often direct, but the women's movement has forced many men to be a little (often not a lot) more subtle. Thus, a decade or so ago, the other members of a poetry workshop at the University of Arizona told me, the only woman there, that my work, though technically brilliant, was—alas—just not very "interesting." (Note the absence of an experiential subject in that judgment. "Interesting to whom?" is not a permissible question.) The same group had gone wild, a couple of meetings before, over another member's poem about his first visit to a whorehouse. I got the message: whorehouses are interesting; wifehood, motherhood, even mistresshood are not.

Beneath questions of "technique" and "interest," I think, lies a deeper issue: control. *Don't construct with your language a version of reality that doesn't square with mine,* the critic is saying. To the poets my technique was fine but my discourse, insofar as it deviated from the principles they had prescribed, was simply not worthy of attention. My reality put them to sleep. I nearly stopped writing for good.

But surely "some of the experiences you describe were at some point superseded when the women's movement came about," a woman chided me after reading an earlier draft of this essay. I'd like to say she's entirely right, but she's not. In college workshops and editorial offices, at writers' conferences and reviewers' desks, women's words continue to be devalued. The fact that the process has grown more exquisite makes it no less pernicious. On the contrary. A stifled yawn of boredom is easily as daunting as a hoot of derision. Some women continue to have experiences similar to mine. Some stop writing, and others resort to depicting not their own experiences but male pornographic fantasies of feminine experience: "Her heart pounding, she pressed her slim, firm, high-breasted body against the length of his lean and muscular frame as her full lips yielded breathlessly to the pressure of his insistent kiss."

But suppose that a woman—thanks indeed to the women's movement—does not stop or swerve? What then can she best do? I would say that she can tell the truth about her body (by which Woolf meant, I'm sure, not just an agglomeration of head and arms and legs and vagina but the embodied self) and its passions, an act which will force her to transgress the boundaries of polite—that is, conventional—discourse, giving tongue to her own delight and desire. That's what I began to do in *Plaintext*, though I didn't know it at the outset; if I had known it, I suspect I'd have been too intimidated to make a peep. At that point I knew only that I'd spent most of my life baffled and in pain over events and feelings that, I was just beginning to sense, weren't peculiar to me. But because they existed in the realm of the linguistically impermissible, I hadn't been able to speak them aloud and, in sharing them with others, ease their weight. I thought that, by writing them down and making them public, I could undermine their power to constrict my life and the lives of any others whose voices had been choked off by social taboos. I think that the key to a happy marriage, as to any sort of happiness, isn't keeping your mouth shut but surfacing and experiencing every bit of life. To do so requires committing life to language, without which nothing recognizable as human can exist.

The life I concocted for myself when I started writing essays turned out to be rather more complicated and ambiguous than the one I had been schooled to receive. It mixed marriage and infidelity, parental love and abandonment, ills of the body and of the heart, the joys of cooking and the habits of cats. Recently, a friend told me that his mother had overheard a conversation in the little book shop in the town where we grew up: "Read it," said a woman, handing *Plaintext* to her companion, "and weep." I don't think it's a sad story, though. I think it's just a *whole* story. And in response to it I began to get letters voicing the feelings of women who had also lived in silence: ". . . a mind cannot be revealed to another and this does cause me anguish. . . . But glimpses of others are possible, I think, and the glimpses you have given me of yourself have helped me feel less afraid and ashamed and alone."

I may sound as though I'm advocating for women's writing merely a kind of therapeutic function: Write two essays and call me in the morning. No. What I think the woman writer should do is the same as what I think the man writer (doesn't that phrase sound funny?) should: make literature, constellations of language that make sense of, and celebrate, what it is to be human. The reason I've been focusing on the woman writer is that I think she still has many experiences, hitherto stifled by convention, to add to that constructive and celebratory process.

We know much about men's experience: they like to fight, to screw, to drink with other men; they are sometimes fonder of their mothers than they think is wholesome; they possess penises, which they think that people without penises should want to possess also; they worship a God who controls them as Father, Lord, Prince, King. We also know what they believe the experiences of women and people of color to be. Now, at last, we've also begun to hear from women and people of color themselves about what it is to them to be human.

We have heard, in a decade of feminism and another of "postfeminism," from many women writers about their lives. Not enough, however. So I think women must go on simply and without apology saying aloud what it is like to be who they are. I've found this difficult myself, both personally and professionally. I've sometimes hurt people I care for, and as a professional I've endured being called a bore (and worse). Mentors and editors have wondered aloud when I'll get around to some "real work," by which they seem to mean something perhaps less personal and certainly less "limited" by feminist perspective.

Still, a major publishing house advanced me enough money to live on while I wrote another book, easily as rude as *Plaintext,* maybe weirder too. The editors there sensed that from the outset. They were willing to share the risk. I worry, though, that such successes will lead me, and women like me, into believing that we are now speaking fully and freely in our own voices "about the body, about the passions," that the women's movement has resolved for good the issues surrounding silence and shame. I worry that complacency will deflect us from the struggle to articulate what remains, to others and to ourselves, unspeakable about our experiences. If we find the work of utterance getting easy or universally acceptable, we're probably not doing it right.

⌒ Faith and Loving in Las Vegas ⌒

If we are to be pilgrims for peace and justice, we must expect the desert.
—DOM HELDER CÁMARA

*L*orenzo is holding my left hand, and Jim is holding my right. Behind me, George holds hands with Jack and Mimi, the three together nudging the wheelchair forward. In the chill, bright desert air our voices float up and mingle with those of the couple of hundred people still behind us:

"Be not afraid. I go before you always. Come, follow Me, and I will give you rest."

A plywood platform has been laid across the wide bars of the cattle guard. The wheelchair bumps up onto the plywood and rolls forward. We have crossed the line.

We are the fourth group to cross. A dozen or more groups will follow us. We are Catholic Workers who have gathered in Las Vegas from all over the country to celebrate the ninetieth anniversary of founder Dorothy Day's birth. We spent yesterday at a Catholic high school in the city, holding workshops and listening to speakers, among them Dom Helder Cámara, the Brazilian archbishop whose labors for the political rights of the poor have transformed the Church throughout the world. He is a figure for whom the simile *birdlike* might have been coined, a tiny aged sparrow of a man in his tan cassock and wooden pectoral cross, his eyes small and bright above dark pouches, his slender fingers gnarled and curved. His accent is thick and his voice is creaky, making his message hard to decipher. But we all understood instantly and cheered when, his right hand inscribing a wide arc above his head, he told us, "We cannot have a First World and a Second World and a Third World and a Fourth World. . . . We must create only One World!"

This morning, Dom Helder among us, we set out from the school in a long caravan across sixty miles of desert, past range after range of humped and spiny mountains, to the Nevada Nuclear Test Site. Beneath this vast sweep of earth, tinted in colors the language has never quite captured (something like rose, like smoke, gray-green, buff), beyond the barbed-wire fence, the United States routinely sets off nuclear explosions, testing what is known already: that We can kill off Them a hundred-fold anytime They step out of line. To protest the deadly provocative desire these explosions signify, some of us have chosen to trespass onto the site, others to blockade access to it with their bodies, still others to line the route and provide support. Although we trespassers are entering federal land, which as taxpayers we have helped to pay for, we are denied any rights in it. We, like the blockaders, know that we will be arrested for our act.

Those of us from Casa María, the Catholic Worker house in Tucson, have clustered together. Despite nearly two decades of social activism, George and I have never committed civil disobedience before, and we are glad to be surrounded by loving and oft-arrested friends. We have been joined for the crossing by Fred and Mimi, a couple in their sixties. Mimi's a writer, and now that he's retired from social work Fred, his polio-damaged legs patched up with steel and Teflon, cooks for the soup kitchen at St. Joseph's on Manhattan's Lower East Side. Once, he's just been telling us, the soup kitchen came into a load of Brie, a dozen or more wheels, and then the hungry and homeless at St. Joseph's got vegetable crêpes with Brie for lunch. The workers found one of the women who lives there seated on her pallet on the floor in her nightgown with a whole wheel of Brie in her lap, gazing far into some other world as she consumed it bite by bite with a teaspoon.

Facing the group of us, the sheriff of Nye County, a slim man with graying temples, says, "First I am going to ask you not to do this." We say nothing. "Then I am going to tell you that if you do it, I will have to arrest you for trespassing." He meets our eyes. "Do you all understand that?"

"Yes," we answer. "Yes, we understand." I don't, I discover, feel as though I'm responding to a question. I feel more the way I do during a baptism, when we break the Nicene Creed into questions and answers: "Do you believe in one God, the Father, the Almighty, Maker of heaven and earth, of all that is seen and unseen?" the priest asks at that time, and the people respond, "I do."

Here, acknowledging that I understand that this weath-ered man with the tired eyes is going to arrest me sounds oddly like a profession of faith.

Deputies begin to handcuff the members of our group. I had envisioned clanking metal circles, the sort that marshals might use to subdue great train robbers, but these are plastic straps like elongated versions of the fas-teners we use to close our trash bags before lugging them out to the alley. I hold my wrists up to be strapped, but the deputy passes me over.

"I'd like to be handcuffed too," I say. My voice sounds ridiculously sedate, as though I'd just asked for two lumps of sugar in my tea. Little did my grandmother suspect, when she drilled me in the tones of a Yankee lady, that I'd find them handy when I got arrested.

"Uh-uh." The deputy shakes his head. "The sher-iff doesn't want you handcuffed." Just then the sheriff looks down at me. "We can't take you in there," he says. "We can't handle a wheelchair on the bus."

"It's all right," I tell him. "Don't worry. I can walk a little. I'll get out of the wheelchair and climb on the bus."

Plainly he's not happy, but he assents.

"My wheelchair," I say. "You will take care of it for me? You won't let anything happen to it, will you?" I haven't for an instant felt afraid of mistreatment by these somber uniformed men, but suddenly I'm scared they might punish me through my wheelchair.

"Don't worry. We'll take good care of it."

It's hard, George discovers, to push a wheelchair across gravel with your hands in cuffs. With Lorenzo, Jim, and Jack helping out, we make a drunken progress toward the bus. Mimi has her cuffed hands full helping Fred, who can't use his Canadian crutch with his hands bound. I don't know how he managed to get handcuffs and I didn't. I suppose it was because he was erect and I was folded up. There is a subtle taxonomy of crippledness.

At the bus I'm glad I don't have handcuffs, though. The steps are very steep, and even holding onto railings on either side, with people in front and back of me for support, I can barely haul myself up. I will be sore for days. Fred has a hard time too, we can see, but he makes it. George and I are given the front seat. He clutches my hand. In a broad-brimmed straw hat and bug-eye sunglasses and a UCLA sweatshirt he looks funny and boyish. "Well," I say, squeezing his hand in return, "this is it. We're across."

Why, I find myself wondering in the first elated rush at being safely on the other side, have we postponed for so long crossing the line between peaceful protest and nonviolent direct action? For me, the progression first from apathy to protest and now from protest to civil disobedience seems hooked somehow to the lives of my children. I crossed that first line in the autumn of 1969, about six months after the birth of my second child, Matthew, when I spotted a full-page advertisement in the *Boston Sunday Globe* protesting the war in Vietnam. Something jolted me then, as it never had before, like a sudden electrical connection: perhaps it was the presence of a small squalling draftable boy whom I was supposed to raise to kill for his country. Whatever the reason, the following day I called the telephone number printed at the bottom of that page.

Thereafter, the small boy and his slightly larger sister riding on our backs and shoulders, George and I began a life of moderate activism. In the intervening years, as the boy and his sister grew astonishingly, we've attended meetings, painted posters, picketed army and air force bases, stood in candlelit vigils. In 1970 we worked to elect an antiwar candidate, the Jesuit priest Robert Drinan, to Congress. We've written letters to editors and legislators. We've boycotted grapes and Campbell products in support of the United Farm Workers. A decade ago, having found a community of people living out their values in ways that inspired us, we converted to Roman Catholicism and later joined Catholics for Peace and Justice. We help to provide food for the hungry, shelter for the homeless, clothing, household equipment, and medical supplies for the poor in Tucson and Central America. To support their economic self-sufficiency, we buy Nicaraguan coffee and crafts made by cooperatives throughout the world. These are worthy enough gestures, and I don't think I'm debasing them by pointing out that they're easy enough as well: they're *safe*. We may encounter—have encountered—familial disapproval and the skepticism of friends. But only rarely have we been physically accosted, and no one has ever threatened to haul us off to jail.

I think that this sense of safety was important to me while I had dependent children. To risk going to jail seemed irresponsible to me while I had to provide for their daily needs. But now Anne has gone off to the Peace

Corps. Matthew, at eighteen, has moved out of the house. In fact, he is struggling just now to decide whether or not to register for the draft. And six months after his eighteenth birthday, here I am in Mercury, Nevada, stepping up my activism, stepping across the next line in my path. Or, in this case, rolling across the next cattle guard.

When the bus is full, we drive a quarter of a mile or so up a straight road, stopping beside a long white trailer. At one end, an area fenced off by posts and wire holds a galvanized metal trash barrel, a couple of white Rent-a-Cans, and the first busloads of the arrested. George and I wait for the others to get off. Just as we are about to follow, a security officer tells me, "You stay right here. We'll ticket you on the bus."

I look at George. I look out the window at the crowd in the pen.

"I don't want to be separated from the others," I say. "I don't want to be left alone. I want to get off the bus."

"There's no place for you to sit." He's right. My wheelchair is back at the crossing.

"I'll sit on the steps," I say. "Or we can turn the trash barrel over and I'll sit on that. I'll sit on one of the toilets. Please. I don't want to be left." The security officer glances at George, who nods, and shrugs. As I head for the steps, the bus driver starts speaking to me softly.

"Do you know what they really do here?" he asks. "They test drugs to help people like you." Actually, no one I know of is working on multiple sclerosis at the atomic level, but I believe that medical research goes on here. "Eighty percent of the testing has nothing to do with weapons."

"It's the twenty percent I'm here about." I find myself speaking softly too. "That's the part that scares me." Some people express anger at his laying such a "trip" on me, but though I'm shocked, I don't feel angry. I feel touched. He's tried to reach out for me as best he can.

I get separated from the others whether I want to or not. A stolid woman in brown trousers and a striped blouse leads me to the steps exiting the trailer, at the opposite end from the holding pen. Those in the pen cheer me as I walk away, and I shrink inwardly in embarrassment. People with whole bodies sometimes mistake cripples for heroes. They forget that I'm doing just what they're doing, only more clumsily. Such self-deprecation denies, however, my real use to them as an emblem of the value of this action. What they are doing is hard. My presence assures them that it is not too hard, that all of us can do whatever we must, here, now, and wherever else we are called. This seems a good enough use to be put to.

Seating me on the gray wooden steps, the woman writes me a ticket for trespassing on federal land "after being advised not to." The fine is $250 plus a $65 processing fee. My court date is December 21, 1987. Some people are giving false identification—many, for this birthday celebration, are being "Dorothy Day"—but I have decided, this time at least, against noncooperation. Naming myself accurately feels like taking responsibility for my act.

When she has finished filling in the blanks and given me my pink copy, she tells me to get back on the bus. I hesitate, looking over at the others. I can't see George.

"Go on," she says. "You can't stay out here. It's not safe."

I am inclined to balk. But, as the sheriff's reluctance to arrest me and my brief interchange with the bus driver have demonstrated, my reality is skewed from the others'. I want to be treated exactly like them. In truth, though, I'm not exactly like them. I'm getting more and more different from them almost by the day. I can't divorce myself, morally or otherwise, from my failing body. I am she. And I have, as a consequence, some responsibilities they can't even grasp. Hell, I can scarcely grasp them myself. All I know is that my crossing the line bears another kind of weight from theirs. It is not a straightforward individual act of civil disobedience. Like it or not, I cross not foremost as a private citizen but as a representative of those people who, despite their disparities, get lumped as the result of their physical disabilities into a single class. Poor people! They haven't asked me to represent them. Most of them would probably shudder at the very idea. But, in a sense, here we all are on a Sunday morning out in the middle of the Nevada desert. Whatever I do will reflect on them.

I feel constrained to be a "good cripple," cheerful and patient, so that whoever might roll along in my wake someday will find the way eased: a stance wholly at odds with the disobedience I am here to practice. I don't know how to resolve this conflict, which has cut me off, quite literally, from the other demonstrators, leaving me as sober and bleak as the landscape I admire from the bus window. The farthest mountain range, bluish and blurred, marks the southern lip of Death Valley, the bus driver explains to me. He is friendly now, maybe conciliatory, though not apologetic.

Slowly the bus is filling. A beautiful young security officer called Bambi jumps up the steps. One of the demonstrators, practicing noncooperation, has given her a hard time, and she's flushed from chasing after him each time he has wandered off toward the desert.

"Which one of you is Dorothy, the one who gave me the cross?" she calls out. The white-haired woman across the aisle from me raises her hand. "I just want to thank you and give you a hug," says Bambi, grinning. "But don't tell anyone I did that or I'll get taken off the line. They know I love this duty so that's how they punish me if I act up. Once they caught me singing and dancing with the people on the bus, and they took me off for *six months.*" We laugh and applaud her.

I wish George were with me. I don't feel alarmed by our separation, as I often do, because I know that everyone here will watch over me until we're back together. In that sense, though I don't know anyone in this group, I'm not among strangers. But I want everything happening here to happen to us together. That's the mark of marriage for me: George's presence roots me more deeply in my own experience. As if my wish had power, he climbs on the bus and hugs me quickly before heading for the last seat, in the back. The doors close, and we turn back to the entrance, stopping there to pick up my wheelchair. If we can put it on the bus now, I don't see why we couldn't have had it with us all along. Oh, well. We are driven back across the line, past the cheering group of demonstrators who have chosen not to be arrested and the silent groups of counterdemonstrators and site workers who are on strike, to the area where we left our cars. George settles me in the wheelchair and, tilting me back, rolls me away from the road. Looking up, I see a white van with the door open, Dom Helder perched on the front seat. I wave to him, and he waves back.

We have made a round trip, across the line and back again, and yet I know that in a way we can never come back. A line, once crossed, can never be *un*crossed. We have, in trespassing, entered new moral terrain, and we will inevitably be transformed in it, though it's too early to tell precisely how. I can glimpse a couple of points already, though. I can tell, for one thing, that I am not the same woman who took up her posters and candles to protest the Vietnam War in 1969. In those days I believed in the efficacy of action. I believed that if I, and others like me, protested emphatically enough, we could sway all right-minded people to our point of view. We could create change. And in a limited way—the only way I started out knowing—I guess I was right. In large measure because of the pressure of popular opinion, the role of the United States in the war in Southeast Asia ground to its ugly and dishonorable close. Perhaps I even believed then that, having learned the error of such ways, the United States would turn utterly from war as a means of structuring human relationships. I was awfully young, remember, not even thirty, and even more ignorant than I am today.

Now I'm not at all sure that I can do anything to prevent the evil—of which nuclear weapons testing, like

CIA covert activities, the trading of arms for hostages, the building of B-1 bombers, the gobbling of federal funds for "defense" rather than the enhancement of human life, is only an emblem—which gnaws at the world's heart. I just don't know. I've come up here to the wilderness to plant my feet on the other side of an invisible line and earn a black mark on my hitherto unbesmirched record without the promise of anything in return. Anything at all.

This terrain seems, at least from where I stand now, foggy and rugged indeed. We are a time-ridden, an ends-addicted society, and no action is valued unless it produces results. By this standard, I have just committed a nonaction. I have just wasted my time. I must be a fool. And yet, smiling foolishly up into Dom Helder's little wrinkled fool's face, I feel certain that something's happening here. I can't change the world. I got lucky once and helped to stop a war, but the world didn't change. The fact that I still confuse Nixon and Reagan is more than a slip of the tongue or the sign of a loose cog somewhere. The men in power, and the women beginning to join them, are, beyond the personal level, indistinguishable: Republican/Democrat, American/Russian, Protestant/Catholic/Muslim/Jew, black/white/yellow/red/brown, all tend to run together. They all thrive on the adrenaline rush triggered by believing one is menaced by An Enemy. They project Enemies right and left to maintain the high. I've got no thrill to offer them to keep their juices pumping like that.

Why, then, do anything at all? If I really believe that no act of mine can break the addiction of those in power, why not lapse into quiescence, accept the world as it is, make the best of a bad thing? Because I have begun to recognize the possibility of relating differently to that world: in the role of witness. I am being transformed by this new understanding from a hot young crusader into a bony finger, pointing: *Here,* the body I have permitted to be arrested testifies, *we are doing wrong. Here we have been unjust. Let's choose another life.* If those in power choose, over my testimony, to blow the world to smithereens instead, I'll be lost with all the rest. I don't believe that right choice confers immunity. I no longer believe in reward. I simply believe that choices must be made regardless of their chances of success. And so I've come here.

The other point I've begun to descry is that although I was arrested for stepping *in*to a giant ring of barbed wire, my true direction is *out*ward. This is not a new movement, of course, but a leap along the trajectory of one I began years ago. I've been shoved and spat on and given the finger—and, in my own more polite circle of family and friends, sighed over—plenty often enough to know that my beliefs do not hold social sway. But my act of civil disobedience has further shrunk the circle of people who understand and share my commitments. I could swagger and say that all others don't matter; but the fact is that they do. Though I don't care much anymore for the world's approval, I yearn for its understanding. Now I've increased the distance between myself and most of the people I come into contact with. They may write me off as a zealot, or a crank. A position on society's margins strengthens one's capacity for the kind of witness I've chosen, I know. All the same, I'm feeling lonely and a little scared. I shiver. George helps me pull on a heavy black sweater and hands me an apple and some almonds.

Late at night, back in Tucson, the weekend's images and insights tumble over and over inside my skull, each turn polishing them to new clarity. In time, I will add them to my hoard. They will travel with me across the next line, and the next. Ahead I've got a lot of moral territory to explore, I know. From where I stand, at the foot of my bed tugging my arms out of my sweater, that territory stretches boundlessly, as shadowy and severe as I imagine the test site to lie at this moment, under tonight's full moon. This sense of vastness both daunts and exhilarates me. In my early activist days, I'm sure I thought that by the time I was forty-four, I'd have all life's ambiguities sorted out and resolved. Now I know that such work goes on forever. To finish it not only isn't possible but—more important—isn't even the point.

"That was a fine experience," I mumble to George through the folds of the nightgown I'm struggling into. "Thank you for pushing me to it, and through it. I guess I can't even get arrested by myself anymore."

"Oh, I don't know." He and the black cat have already snugged down under the covers, and his voice is muffled by blankets and sleep. "Knowing you the way I do, I think you'd manage to find some way to get arrested on your own."

Doubtless he's right. But why, after all, would I want to? Getting arrested, like any of life's necessary tasks, is eased and enriched by company. And one cannot make the world's peace, by its very nature, in solitude.

Peace must be woven intentionally, meticulously, clasped hand by clasped hand, across all the desert spaces between us.

Holdings hands, with the black cat tucked between us, George and I sleep.

⌒ Carnal Acts ⌒

*I*nviting me to speak at her small liberal-arts college during Women's Week, a young woman set me a task: "We would be pleased," she wrote, "if you could talk on how you cope with your M.S. disability, and also how you discovered your voice as a writer." Oh, Lord, I thought in dismay, how am I going to pull this one off? How can I yoke two such disparate subjects into a coherent presentation, without doing violence to one, or the other, or both, or myself? This is going to take some fancy footwork, and my feet scarcely carry out the basic steps, let alone anything elaborate.

To make matters worse, the assumption underlying each of her questions struck me as suspect. To ask *how* I cope with multiple sclerosis suggests that I *do* cope. Now, "to cope," *Webster's Third* tells me, is "to face or encounter and to find necessary expedients to overcome problems and difficulties." In these terms, I have to confess, I don't feel like much of a coper. I'm likely to deal with my problems and difficulties by squawking and flapping around like that hysterical chicken who was convinced the sky was falling. Never mind that in my case the sky really *is* falling. In response to a clonk on the head, regardless of its origin, one might comport oneself with a grace and courtesy I generally lack.

As for "finding" my voice, the implication is that it was at one time lost or missing. But I don't think it ever was. Ask my mother, who will tell you a little wearily that I was speaking full sentences by the time I was a year old and could never be silenced again. As for its being a writer's voice, it seems to have become one early on. Ask Mother again. At the age of eight I rewrote the Trojan War, she will say, and what Nestor was about to do to Helen at the end doesn't bear discussion in polite company.

Faced with these uncertainties, I took my own teacherly advice, something, I must confess, I don't always do. "If an idea is giving you trouble," I tell my writing students, "put it on the back burner and let it simmer while you do something else. Go to the movies. Reread a stack of old love letters. Sit in your history class and take detailed notes on the Teapot Dome scandal. If you've got your idea in mind, it will go on cooking at some level no matter what else you're doing." "I've had an idea for my documented essay on the back burner," one of my students once scribbled in her journal, "and I think it's just boiled over!"

I can't claim to have reached such a flash point. But

in the weeks I've had the themes "disability" and "voice" sitting around in my head, they seem to have converged on their own, without my having to wrench them together and bind them with hoops of tough rhetoric. They *are* related, indeed interdependent, with an intimacy that has for some reason remained, until now, submerged below the surface of my attention. Forced to juxtapose them, I yank them out of the depths, a little startled to discover how they were intertwined down there out of sight. This kind of discovery can unnerve you at first. You feel like a giant hand that, pulling two swimmers out of the water, two separate heads bobbling on the iridescent swells, finds the two bodies below, legs coiled around each other, in an ecstasy of copulation. You don't quite know where to turn your eyes.

Perhaps the place to start illuminating this erotic connection between who I am and how I speak lies in history. I have known that I have multiple sclerosis for about seventeen years now, though the disease probably started long before. The hypothesis is that the disease process, in which the protective covering of the nerves in the brain and spinal cord is eaten away and replaced by scar tissue, "hard patches," is caused by an autoimmune reaction to a slow-acting virus. Research suggests that I was infected by this virus, which no one has ever seen and which therefore, technically, doesn't even "exist," between the ages of four and fifteen. In effect, living with this mysterious mechanism feels like having your present self, and the past selves it embodies, haunted by a capricious and meanspirited ghost, unseen except for its footprints, which trips you even when you're watching where you're going, knocks glassware out of your hand, squeezes the urine out of your bladder before you reach the bathroom, and weights your whole body with a weariness no amount of rest can relieve. An alien invader must be at work. But of course it's not. It's your own body. That is, it's you.

This, for me, has been the most difficult aspect of adjusting to a chronic incurable degenerative disease: the fact that it has rammed my "self" straight back into the body I had been trained to believe it could, through high-minded acts and aspirations, rise above. The Western tradition of distinguishing the body from the mind and/or the soul is so ancient as to have become part of our collective unconscious, if one is inclined to believe in such a noumenon, or at least to have become an unquestioned element in the social instruction we impose upon infants from birth, in much the same way we inculcate, without reflection, the gender distinctions "female" and "male." I *have* a body, you are likely to say if you talk about embodiment at all; you don't say, I *am* a body. A body is a separate entity possessable by the "I"; the "I" and the body aren't, as the copula would make them, grammatically indistinguishable.

To widen the rift between the self and the body, we treat our bodies as subordinates, inferior in moral status. Open association with them shames us. In fact, we treat our bodies with very much the same distance and ambivalence women have traditionally received from men in our culture. Sometimes this treatment is benevolent, even respectful, but all too often it is tainted by outright sadism. I think of the bodybuilding regimens that have become popular in the last decade or so, with the complicated vacillations they reflect between self-worship and self-degradation: joggers and aerobic dancers and weightlifters all beating their bodies into shape. "No pain, no gain," the saying goes. "Feel the burn." Bodies get treated like wayward women who have to be shown who's boss, even if it means slapping them around a little. I'm not for a moment opposing rugged exercise here. I'm simply questioning the spirit in which it is often undertaken.

Since, as Hélène Cixous points out in her essay on women and writing, "Sorties,"* thought has always worked "through dual, hierarchical oppositions" (p. 64), the mind/body split cannot possibly be innocent. The utterance of an "I" immediately calls into being its opposite, the "not-I," Western discourse being unequipped to conceive "that which is neither 'I' nor 'not-I,' " "that which is both 'I' and 'not-I,' " or some other permutation which language doesn't permit me to speak. The "not-I" is, by definition, other. And we've never been too fond of the other. We prefer the same. We tend to ascribe to the other those qualities we prefer not to associate with our selves: it is the hidden, the dark, the secret, the shameful. Thus, when the "I" takes possession of the body, it makes the body into an other, direct object of a transitive verb, with all the other's repudiated and potentially dangerous qualities.

At the least, then, the body had best be viewed

*In *The Newly Born Woman*, translated by Betsy Wing (Minneapolis: University of Minnesota Press, 1986).

with suspicion. And a woman's body is particularly suspect, since so much of it is in fact hidden, dark, secret,
carried about on the inside where, even with the aid of a
speculum, one can never perceive all of it in the plain light
of day, a graspable whole. I, for one, have never understood why anyone would want to carry all that delicate
stuff around on the outside. It would make you awfully
anxious, I should think, put you constantly on the defen-
sive, create a kind of siege mentality that viewed all other
beings, even your own kind, as threats to be warded off
with spears and guns and atomic missiles. And you'd
never get to experience that inward dreaming that comes
when your flesh surrounds all your treasures, holding
them close, like a sturdy shuttered house. Be my personal
skepticism as it may, however, as a cultural woman I bear
just as much shame as any woman for my dark, enfolded
secrets. Let the word for my external genitals tell the tale:
my pudendum, from the Latin infinitive meaning "to be
ashamed."

It's bad enough to carry your genitals like a sealed
envelope bearing the cipher that, once unlocked, might
loose the chaotic flood of female pleasure—*jouissance,* the
French call it—upon the world-of-the-same. But I have
an additional reason to feel shame for my body, less ex-
plicitly connected with its sexuality: it is a crippled body.
Thus it is doubly other, not merely by the homo-sexual
standards of patriarchal culture but by the standards of
physical desirability erected for every body in our world.
Men, who are by definition exonerated from shame in
sexual terms (this doesn't mean that an individual man
might not experience sexual shame, of course; remember

that I'm talking in general about discourse, not folks), may—more likely must—experience bodily shame if they are crippled. I won't presume to speak about the details of their experience, however. I don't know enough. I'll just go on telling what it's like to be a crippled woman, trusting that, since we're fellow creatures who've been living together for some thousands of years now, much of my experience will resonate with theirs.

I was never a beautiful woman, and for that reason I've spent most of my life (together with probably at least 95 percent of the female population of the United States) suffering from the shame of falling short of an unattainable standard. The ideal woman of my generation was . . . perky, I think you'd say, rather than gorgeous. Blond hair pulled into a bouncing ponytail. Wide blue eyes, a turned-up nose with maybe a scattering of golden freckles across it, a small mouth with full lips over straight white teeth. Her breasts were large but well harnessed high on her chest; her tiny waist flared to hips just wide enough to give the crinolines under her circle skirt a starting outward push. In terms of personality, she was outgoing, even bubbly, not pensive or mysterious. Her milieu was the front fender of a white Corvette convertible, surrounded by teasing crewcuts, dressed in black flats, a sissy blouse, and the letter sweater of the Corvette owner. Needless to say, she never missed a prom.

Ten years or so later, when I first noticed the symptoms that would be diagnosed as MS, I was probably looking my best. Not beautiful still, but the ideal had shifted enough so that my flat chest and narrow hips gave me an elegantly attenuated shape, set off by a thick mass of long, straight, shining hair. I had terrific legs, long and shapely, revealed nearly to the pudendum by the fashionable miniskirts and hot pants I adopted with more enthusiasm than delicacy of taste. Not surprisingly, I suppose, during this time I involved myself in several pretty torrid love affairs.

The beginning of MS wasn't too bad. The first symptom, besides the pernicious fatigue that had begun to devour me, was "foot drop," the inability to raise my left foot at the ankle. As a consequence, I'd started to limp, but I could still wear high heels, and a bit of a limp might seem more intriguing than repulsive. After a few months, when the doctor suggested a cane, a crippled friend gave me quite an elegant wood-and-silver one, which I carried with a fair amount of panache. The real blow to my self-image came when I had to get a brace. As braces go, it's not bad: lightweight plastic molded to my foot and leg, fitting down into an ordinary shoe and secured around my calf by a Velcro strap. It reduces my limp and, more important, the danger of tripping and falling. But it meant the end of high heels. And it's ugly. Not as ugly as I think it is, I gather, but still pretty ugly. It signified for me, and perhaps still does, the permanence and irreversibility of my condition. The brace makes my MS concrete and forces me to wear it on the outside. As soon as I strapped the brace on, I climbed into trousers and stayed there (though not in the same trousers, of course). The idea of going around with my bare brace hanging out seemed almost as indecent as exposing my breasts. Not until 1984, soon after I won the Western States Book Award for poetry, did I put on a skirt short enough to reveal my plasticized leg. The connection between winning a writing award and baring my brace is not merely fortuitous; being affirmed as a writer really did embolden me. Since then, I've grown so accustomed to wearing skirts that I don't think about my brace any more than I think about my cane. I've incorporated them, I suppose: made them, in their necessity, insensate but fundamental parts of my body.

Meanwhile, I had to adjust to the most outward and visible sign of all, a three-wheeled electric scooter called an Amigo. This lessens my fatigue and increases my range terrifically, but it also shouts out to the world, "Here is a woman who can't stand on her own two feet." At the same time, paradoxically, it renders me invisible, reducing me to the height of a seven-year-old, with a child's attendant low status. "Would she like smoking or nonsmoking?" the gate agent assigning me a seat asks the friend traveling with me. In crowds I see nothing but buttocks. I can tell you the name of every type of designer jeans ever sold. The wearers, eyes front, trip over me and fall across my handlebars into my lap. "Hey!" I want to shout to the lofty world. "Down here! There's a person down here!" But I'm not, by their standards, quite a person anymore.

My self-esteem diminishes further as age and illness strip from me the features that made me, for a brief while anyway, a good-looking, even sexy, young woman. No more long, bounding strides: I shuffle along with the timid gait I remember observing, with pity and impatience, in the little old ladies at Boston's Symphony Hall on Friday afternoons. No more lithe, girlish figure: my belly sags from the loss of muscle tone, which also creates all kinds of intestinal disruptions, hopelessly humiliating in a society in which excretory functions remain strictly unspeakable. No more sex, either, if society had its way. The sexuality of the disabled so repulses most people that you can hardly get a doctor, let alone a member of the general population, to consider the issues it raises. Cripples simply aren't supposed to Want It, much less Do It. Fortunately, I've got a husband with a strong libido and a weak sense of social propriety, or else I'd find myself perforce practicing a vow of chastity I never cared to take.

Afflicted by the general shame of having a body at all, and the specific shame of having one weakened and misshapen by disease, I ought not to be able to hold my head up in public. And yet I've gotten into the habit of holding my head up in public, sometimes under excruciating circumstances. Recently, for instance, I had to give a reading at the University of Arizona. Having smashed three of my front teeth in a fall onto the concrete floor of my screened porch, I was in the process of getting them crowned, and the temporary crowns flew out during dinner right before the reading. What to do? I wanted, of course, to rush home and hide till the dental office opened the next morning. But I couldn't very well break my word at this last moment. So, looking like Hansel and Gretel's witch, and lisping worse than the Wife of Bath, I got up on stage and read. Somehow, over the years, I've learned how to set shame aside and do what I have to do.

Here, I think, is where my "voice" comes in. Because, in spite of my demurral at the beginning, I do in fact cope with my disability at least some of the time. And

I do so, I think, by speaking about it, and about the whole experience of being a body, specifically a female body, out loud, in a clear, level tone that drowns out the frantic whispers of my mother, my grandmothers, all the other trainers of wayward childish tongues: "Sssh! Sssh! Nice girls don't talk like that. Don't mention sweat. Don't mention menstrual blood. Don't ask what your grandfather does on his business trips. Don't laugh so loud. You sound like a loon. Keep your voice down. Don't tell. Don't tell. Don't tell." Speaking out loud is an antidote to shame. I want to distinguish clearly here between "shame," as I'm using the word, and "guilt" and "embarrassment," which, though equally painful, are not similarly poisonous. Guilt arises from performing a forbidden act or failing to perform a required one. In either case, the guilty person can, through reparation, erase the offense and start fresh. Embarrassment, less opprobrious though not necessarily less distressing, is generally caused by acting in a socially stupid or awkward way. When I trip and sprawl in public, when I wet myself, when my front teeth fly out, I feel horribly embarrassed, but, like the pain of childbirth, the sensation blurs and dissolves in time. If it didn't, every child would be an only child, and no one would set foot in public after the onset of puberty, when embarrassment erupts like a geyser and bathes one's whole life in its bitter stream. Shame may attach itself to guilt or embarrassment, complicating their resolution, but it is not the same emotion. I feel guilt or embarrassment for something I've done; shame, for who I am. I may stop doing bad or stupid things, but I can't stop being. How then can I help but be ashamed? Of the three conditions, this is the one that cracks and stifles my voice.

I can subvert its power, I've found, by acknowledging who I am, shame and all, and, in doing so, raising what was hidden, dark, secret about my life into the plain light of shared human experience. What we aren't permitted to utter holds us, each isolated from every other, in a kind of solipsistic thrall. Without any way to check our reality against anyone else's, we assume that our fears and shortcomings are ours alone. One of the strangest consequences of publishing a collection of personal essays called *Plaintext* has been the steady trickle of letters and telephone calls saying essentially, in a tone of unmistakable relief, "Oh, me too! Me too!" It's as though the part I thought was solo has turned out to be a chorus. But none of us was singing loud enough for the others to hear.

Singing loud enough demands a particular kind of voice, I think. And I was wrong to suggest, at the beginning, that I've always had my voice. I have indeed always had *a* voice, but it wasn't *this* voice, the one with which I could call up and transform my hidden self from a naughty girl into a woman talking directly to others like herself. Recently, in the process of writing a new book, a memoir entitled *Remembering the Bone House*, I've had occasion to read some of my early writing, from college, high school, even junior high. It's not an experience I recommend to anyone susceptible to shame. Not that the writing was all that bad. I was surprised at how competent a lot of it was. Here was a writer who already knew precisely how the language worked. But the voice . . . oh, the voice was all wrong: maudlin, rhapsodic, breaking here and there into little shrieks, almost, you might say, hysterical. It was a voice that had shucked off its own body, its own homely life of Cheerios for breakfast and seventy pages of Chaucer to read before the exam on Tuesday and a planter's wart growing painfully on the ball of its foot, and reeled now wraithlike through the air, seeking incarnation only as the heroine who enacts her doomed love for the tall, dark, mysterious stranger. If it didn't get that part, it wouldn't play at all.

Among all these overheated and vaporous imaginings, I must have retained some shred of sense, because I stopped writing prose entirely, except for scholarly papers, for nearly twenty years. I even forgot, not exactly that I had written prose, but at least what kind of prose it was. So when I needed to take up the process again, I could start almost fresh, using the vocal range I'd gotten used to in years of asking the waiter in the Greek restaurant for an extra anchovy on my salad, congratulating the puppy on making a puddle outside rather than inside the patio door, pondering with my daughter the vagaries of female orgasm, saying goodbye to my husband, and hello, and goodbye, and hello. This new voice—thoughtful, affectionate, often amused—was essential because what I needed to write about when I returned to prose was an attempt I'd made not long before to kill myself, and suicide simply refuses to be spoken of authentically in high-flown romantic language. It's too ugly. Too shameful. Too strictly a bodily event. And, yes, too funny as well, though people are sometimes shocked to find humor shoved up against suicide. They don't like the incongruity. But let's face it, life (real life, I mean, not the edited-for-television version) is a cacophonous affair from start to finish. I might have wanted to portray my suicidal self as a languishing maiden, too exquisitely sensitive to sustain life's wounding pressures on her soul. (I didn't want to, as a matter of fact, but I might have.) The truth remained, regardless of my desires, that when my husband lugged me into the emergency room, my hair matted, my face swollen and gray, my nightgown streaked with blood and urine, I was no frail and tender spirit. I was a body, and one in a hell of a mess.

I "should" have kept quiet about that experience. I know the rules of polite discourse. I should have kept my shame, and the nearly lethal sense of isolation and alienation it brought, to myself. And I might have, except for something the psychiatrist in the emergency room had told my husband. "You might as well take her home," he said. "If she wants to kill herself, she'll do it no matter how many precautions we take. They always do." *They* always do. I was one of "them," whoever they were. I was, in this context anyway, not singular, not aberrant, but typical. I think it was this sense of commonality with others I didn't even know, a sense of being returned somehow, in spite of my appalling act, to the human family, that urged me to write that first essay, not merely speaking out but calling out, perhaps. "Here's the way I am," it said. "How about you?" And the answer came, as I've said: "Me too! Me too!"

This has been the kind of work I've continued to do: to scrutinize the details of my own experience and to report what I see, and what I think about what I see, as lucidly and accurately as possible. But because feminine

experience has been immemorially devalued and repressed, I continue to find this task terrifying. "Every
woman has known the torture of beginning to speak
aloud," Cixous writes, "heart beating as if to break, occasionally falling into loss of language, ground and language
slipping out from under her, because for woman speaking—even just opening her mouth—in public is something rash, a transgression" (p. 92).

The voice I summon up wants to crack, to whisper,
to trail back into silence. "I'm sorry to have nothing more
than this to say," it wants to apologize. "I shouldn't be
taking up your time. I've never fought in a war, or even
in a schoolyard free-for-all. I've never tried to see who
could piss farthest up the barn wall. I've never even been
to a whorehouse. All the important formative experiences
have passed me by. I was raped once. I've borne two
children. Milk trickling out of my breasts, blood trickling
from between my legs. You don't want to hear about it.
Sometimes I'm too scared to leave my house. Not scared
of anything, just scared: mouth dry, bowels writhing.
When the fear got really bad, they locked me up for six
months, but that was years ago. I'm getting old now.
Misshapen, too. I don't blame you if you can't get it up.
No one could possibly desire a body like this. It's not your
fault. It's mine. Forgive me. I didn't mean to start crying.
I'm sorry . . . sorry . . . sorry. . . ."

An easy solace to the anxiety of speaking aloud:
this slow subsidence beneath the waves of shame, back
into what Cixous calls "this body that has been worse than
confiscated, a body replaced with a disturbing stranger,
sick or dead, who so often is a bad influence, the cause and

place of inhibitions. By censuring the body," she goes on, "breath and speech are censored at the same time" (p. 97). But I am not going back, not going under one more time. To do so would demonstrate a failure of nerve far worse than the depredations of MS have caused. Paradoxically, losing one sort of nerve has given me another. No one is going to take my breath away. No one is going to leave me speechless. To be silent is to comply with the standard of feminine grace. But my crippled body already violates all notions of feminine grace. What more have I got to lose? I've gone beyond shame. I'm shameless, you might say. You know, as in "shameless hussy"? A woman with her bare brace and her tongue hanging out.

I've "found" my voice, then, just where it ought to have been, in the body-warmed breath escaping my lungs and throat. Forced by the exigencies of physical disease to embrace my self in the flesh, I couldn't write bodiless prose. The voice is the creature of the body that produces it. I speak as a crippled woman. At the same time, in the utterance I redeem both "cripple" and "woman" from the shameful silences by which I have often felt surrounded, contained, set apart; I give myself permission to live openly among others, to reach out for them, stroke them with fingers and sighs. No body, no voice; no voice, no body. That's what I know in my bones.

↪ Challenge: An Exploration ↩

*I*n recent months I've had to give a good bit of thought to the concept of challenge because I have, in the venerable tradition of explorers, stepped off the edge of my known world and have encountered, in the wilderness beyond, numerous tests of my stamina and pluck. "Go west, middle-aged woman" came the call, and I responded by accepting the offer of a lectureship in the UCLA Writing Programs. Since my husband and son had responsibilities in Tucson, and my daughter was finishing her senior year at Smith College, in quite the opposite direction, I had to set off on my venture alone.

I'm not accustomed to venturing out alone. In our twenty-odd years of marriage, George and I have almost always been together, most of that time accompanied by children and assorted sojourners and a series of cats remarkable for its length and diversity: the Mino, Ho Tei,

Ho's Anna, Kitten Little, the Princess Saralinda, Katy, Balthasar, Mimi, Freya, Gwydion, Burton Rustle, Bête Noire, Vanessa Bell, Lionel Tigress, Eclipse, and most recently a wicked little black scrap called Sophia and her brother Sebastian. And for well over half that time, I've been increasingly crippled by multiple sclerosis. Thus, not only was I uncertain that I could be content without human and feline companionship; I wasn't even sure that I could take care of myself and my household of one on my own. But there didn't seem to be any safe way of finding out. I'd simply have to do it and watch what happened.

Our plan was to give me as well-supported a start as possible. During the summer I accumulated the goods it seemed I'd need: some just for fun, like a little television, and others purely practical, like a hand-held electric can opener and a collapsible shopping cart for trundling groceries and laundry. These we would load into my aging Volvo station wagon, and on the eighteenth of September George would drive me across the desert and settle me in the small apartment I'd rented.

Then life did what life so often does to mice and men. Three days before our scheduled departure came the telephone call one always dreads: George's father had died, quickly and without suffering, that afternoon at his home in Vermont. Suddenly all our plans seemed meaningless. All that mattered was to get George onto a plane immediately for an indefinite trip East.

But I was committed to the westward journey. My duties would begin in a week. And so I unpacked my boxes and repacked what I could squeeze into a couple of suitcases and a couple of carry-on bags and flew to Los Angeles on the day we had planned to arrive, prepared to camp out in my apartment until George could bring me my car and household goods. At the airport I rented a zippy little red Nova and set out through the streets of Los Angeles (the freeways, I knew, were beyond any bravery I had ever summoned, and in fact I have yet to set wheel upon them) to locate my new home. And I did! Foolish with elation, I pulled up in front of a block-long white apartment building in one corner of which, as though among the Anasazi at Mesa Verde, I would crouch in my own small space. A colleague from the Writing Programs and his wife lived there too, and with their help I unloaded the car, bought some groceries, and began to settle in.

I was exhausted but pretty pleased with myself. I was taking on tasks I'd never dreamed I could handle, not just moving to Los Angeles but even arranging the whole procedure myself. In a Greek tragedy, my self-congratulation would be known as *hubris,* and the chorus would make plain to you that my downfall was inevitable. According to the cautionary puritanical wisdom of my Yankee youth, "Pride goeth before a fall." Note that both visions of the human lot share the image of collapse.

I fell flat on my face. Literally. About thirty hours after my arrival, as I stepped off the elevator into my garage, I tripped and pitched forward, striking my head on the concrete floor. When I came to, the face of a paramedic hovered near my eyes, a circle of dimmer, curious faces floating beyond.

"I'm so frightened," I said.

"Don't worry," said the paramedic as he settled

me onto a stretcher. "You're going to be just fine." Perhaps he says that to everyone, the laboring woman and the black boy with the bullet in his butt and the security guard pummeled by a thief, all of whom I saw in the emergency room at Brotman Medical Center that night. No doubt paramedics specialize in the power of positive thinking rather than actual prognostication. At any rate, in my case he was right. I got x-rayed and stitched up and spent a couple of days under observation in an extra bed in the Michael Jackson Burn Center and was sent home, looking just as though someone had rammed a California plum into my left eye socket, in time to make the second day of orientation at UCLA, where I worked for the following six months, on a campus just about as ill-suited to the needs and limitations of the physically disabled as you can imagine: steps everywhere, parking spaces nowhere, slippery brick sidewalks, women's rooms on every other floor, elevator doors that snap quicker than Godzilla's jaws.

In the context of all these upheavals and adjustments, during which I spent all but a few hours each week alone, I meditated at length on challenge: What it is. What it's good for. Whether I want anything at all to do with it.

Recently I've become aware of a new euphemism for the disabled (which is itself, if not a euphemism, at least a designation so abstract as to be nearly meaningless): the "physically challenged." I don't like euphemisms, which constitute a verbal trick for pretending that what is real and sometimes ugly about our lives isn't happening, or is happening but "really" isn't so bad, or that what is happening in our lives is for the best, maybe even for our own good. I don't think any of those thoughts about my multiple sclerosis or my sixteen-year-old niece's blindness or any other radical loss or limitation. For this reason, as I've pointed out elsewhere, I call myself a cripple. I do so because the word is the most accurate and precise I've found, meaning that I no longer have full use of my limbs. That's all it means, by the way (look it up in your dictionary), and I'm not really clear where all the emotional baggage people toss onto it comes from. But in contemporary society the baggage is there for "cripple," as it is for "death" (people aren't permitted simply to die: they "pass on" or "away," "go to their just reward," or "enter into heaven," though maybe they no longer sleep, like the Victorians, "in the arms of Morpheus"). And I think the squeamishness about the two words is related. We really don't want to confront the radical transformations of our bodies.

Hence a phrase like "physically challenged," which struck me as pure bellywash from the moment I heard it over the telephone last spring from a pleasant MS person in California who'd just read an excerpt from my book *Plaintext.* "You shouldn't call yourself a cripple," she remonstrated. "In our group we refer to ourselves as the physically challenged. It suggests a much healthier attitude." I believe people have the right to call themselves whatever they please. And I'm all for healthy attitudes. Lord knows mine gets pretty peaked much of the time. But I don't think a cure for its anemia is a dose of language like "physically challenged" for the simple reason that I have no idea what that phrase means. (I didn't ask my caller, but I supposed one might by analogy call someone

101

with Alzheimer's or Down's syndrome "mentally challenged," with the same fuzzy results; and sure enough, a few weeks ago I came across just that phrase.) The purpose of a word is to identify a phenomenon precisely and distinguish it from all other phenomena. And though, when I'm faced with one of the pigeon-toed shopping carts at the Safeway which, with all my strength, I can barely wrestle up one aisle and down the next, I *know* that I'm physically challenged, I don't see how that phrase distinguishes me from anyone else who works hard or plays hard—from, say, the latest climber struggling up the face of Mount Everest. And, lurching along from ice cream to paper towels, *I am different* from that woman in her parka and goggles, face cracked and blackened, setting out on the last day's exhausted plod to the summit. Not better, or worse, but different. And I have to recognize that difference, not disguise it, in order to live authentically, that is, according to my true self.

So I toss aside "physically challenged" on the grounds that it enables me to pretend that difference doesn't matter. But I have another and more urgent reason as well. We are living, rock star Madonna reminds us, in a material world, and we're all material boys and girls. As a society we are obsessively attached, thanks largely to slick advertising campaigns with budgets big enough to feed entire countries for years, to the emblems of sheer physicality: to BMWs and powerful stereo systems and Big Macs with fries and movies every Saturday night and above all to our bodies, which we starve and roast and stretch and pummel and sanitize (deodorant, toothpaste, mouthwash, shampoo, cologne . . .) in a frenetic attempt to "make statements" about ourselves, we say, to let the world know who we are, as though identity really rode in a BMW or flaunted bronzed skin.

I hear in "physically challenged" the same sort of emphasis, the concern with the body's tasks, its difficulties, its accomplishments. These are real, God knows. But I'm not sure they're particularly important. I admit that I have squandered a vast deal of energy and attention doddering from my apartment door to the chute at the end of the hall and maneuvering a bulging plastic sack of Coke cans and old newspapers into the stinking hole, but I don't believe that what I do with my trash is an intrinsically interesting question. What I do with my inward being—with the woman raging at her own wastefulness and weakness, terrified of losing her balance, lonely for her husband who has always made her trash disappear before—that's a different matter, a matter of some urgency, I think. How we respond to physical demands, all of us—Nancy at the Safeway and the woman crouched on the escarpment in the shadow of Mount Everest's summit, everyone reading this essay, whether "disabled" or not, our loved ones, our enemies—and what choices we make in the face of danger, and difficulty, and loss determine the true shape and depth of our being. I think of us all as "spiritually challenged." I think of spiritual challenge as the human condition.

Perhaps those of us who are disabled enjoy some advantages in this area—some special knowledge about coping with adversity, for instance. I can't really say. To do so might lead to some form of silly one-upmanship of the spirit ("my condition is more spiritually challenging than your condition"). But I can say that disability provides ample opportunity for spiritual work and growth. Those of us with degenerative diseases must learn to accommodate uncertainty equably, for instance, and to make our plans for the future as leaps of faith rather than sure bets. We must practice patience with the general populace of "temporarily abled persons," who often seem to us as heedless as children. We must learn—a task particularly difficult for women, I find—to articulate our needs clearly and insist on our rights to treatment that enables us to function most fully; but we must also learn not to ask for more than we need out of the typical human weakness for ease at any price. We must accept responsibility for ourselves and our own well-being, and we mustn't give up too readily the difficult tasks we set ourselves. But—a truth I am only beginning to confront as my right side, always my "good" side, quickly weakens— we must also be willing to let go gracefully of tasks that have become impossible, with as little anger and self-recrimination as possible.

Anyone who can accomplish such feats—and the many more that disability demands—will be a saint indeed. Myself, I don't know anyone who's come even close. But sainthood isn't really my concern. Just challenge, and our responses to it. And I say, let's not hide behind meaningless phrases in an attempt to fool ourselves that our lives are somehow easier than they are; let's look at our lives as squarely, and as lovingly, as we can. And let's not be deflected by concerns about our bodies, their images and their illnesses, from what is most significant about our selves: that we can grow in courage, in grit, in spirit, not in spite of who we are but because of who we are.

Doing It the Hard Way

Not long ago, my daughter graduated from Smith College, a liberal arts college for women in Massachusetts, along with nearly seven hundred classmates. Many of the graduates were already poised to plunge into worlds of prestige and wealth, on Wall Street or Madison Avenue or Capitol Hill, glittering with the promise of a life of ease: a condo with a river view, a silver BMW convertible, summer vacations on the coast of Maine and winter vacations in Barbados. Others, deferring these rewards, planned first to attend medical school, law school, business school. And some, wavering in the face of the choices a privileged education proffers, when asked about their plans replied with comic defensiveness, "I don't know, and I don't care, so don't ask!"

Because Anne had majored in biochemistry, most people assumed that she'd go to medical school or get a

Ph.D. and become a research scientist. But she's never showed a glimmer of interest in doctoring human beings, though in high school she did contemplate becoming a veterinarian and even spent a few weeks in Honduras vaccinating pigs against hog cholera. She gave some thought to training as a pharmacist, but she was heartily sick of school. Instead, she chose a course of action that surprised even those of us closest to her: she joined the Peace Corps.

Now she lives, with a tabby kitten named Nuni, in a house at one end of the village of Mfuatu in western Zaïre. Nobody there speaks English, but she's picking up French and Kikongo, though when she was nursing herself through an attack of malaria recently, her attempts at explaining the use of a fever thermometer to the children who trail after her wherever she goes merely baffled everyone involved in the broken dialogue. Every morning she bathes with the other women in a nearby river, returning with enough water for the day's needs. During the day, she rides the dirt roads of her area on a Yamaha 125 motorcycle, visiting local farmers to teach them how to build ponds, stock them with tilapia, and maintain and harvest the fish to feed themselves and to sell for income. At night, by candle or kerosene lamp, she writes us letters that reflect a complicated mixture of distress and delight at her new life.

When she decided to go, her father and I were thrilled, but she encountered some resistance and even more incomprehension from some of her family and friends. Why would anyone, they wanted to know, especially a young woman as bright and promising as Anne, go off to spend two years in poverty, without even electricity or plumbing, eating a diet that has included grasshoppers and snakes, exposed to deadly diseases like yellow fever and cholera without a doctor for miles of rutted road that turns to muddy soup with every rain? What about the handsome salary, the condo, the BMW, not to mention the eligible young electrical engineer eager to make her his wife?

I'm not sure why. Anne tends to keep her own counsel, and she was too scared to talk much about her choice the summer before she left. But I don't think she was repudiating graduate school or big paychecks, or even condos and BMWs. She may well want them when she returns. They just didn't seem to be enough. I think she went in part to postpone momentous decisions about marriage and career until she knew more about herself and the world. She's always been a woman of action, not words, and the Peace Corps offered her the chance to experience the lives of others directly and help them meet their own needs, not the needs some ideologue might believe they ought to feel. But mostly, I gathered from what little she had to say, she went for the adventure, and the personal growth that carrying out difficult tasks stimulates. Materially privileged and intellectually gifted, she'd never come close to her limits, and I think she wanted to put her capacities to the test. When I hear excitement and satisfaction in the tone of her letters, I find myself thinking, "At last she's found something hard enough for her."

Most people don't have to light out for Africa in order to seek out a difficult life. Indeed, some of us have difficulty plump itself right into our laps without so much as a by-your-leave. I'm going to speak in terms of having multiple sclerosis, because this incurable neurological disease is the difficulty that barged into my life uninvited. But if difficulty doesn't arrive as MS, sooner or later it arrives in some form: the lost job, the child gone wrong, the parent with Alzheimer's, the marriage truncated by death or divorce. And then we have to choose how we will respond to the "gift" of a difficult life.

Anne's adventure, and the sense I have that somehow the hardships she's chosen to endure in order to have that adventure are integral to the adventure's value, have led me to reflect at length on the whole matter of "difficulty." It is, I've come to see, something of a dirty word in our society. "Take it easy," we tell one another at the first sign of agitation. "Kick back and relax." "Don't get your liver in a quiver." A hard life isn't any fun. The good life, the media relentlessly drum into our eyes and ears, is the one that takes the least effort. We develop laborsaving devices to help achieve it, sometimes even labeling them to convey the essence of their desirability: my mother had an "Easy" washer and dryer for years, for instance. "Why do things the hard way?" we ask.

If our lives do prove difficult, troublesome, even painful, we're reluctant to admit it. To experience difficulty suggests some sort of weakness, and to admit to experiencing difficulty risks accusations of whining and self-pity. In either case, we feel shame. I discovered just how pervasive this reaction is when my husband asked me what I was at work on currently.

"I'm writing about the ways people respond to a difficult life," I told him.

"Oh, well," George said, as though in response to a question I hadn't even asked, "*I* don't have a difficult life." Now, this is a man who has raised three children, one of them a foster child; who has assisted a wife with multiple sclerosis for more than fifteen years; who has had two melanomas surgically removed; who holds two jobs, both teaching students who have failed in conventional settings. These are all, without question, both physically and mentally arduous undertakings. And yet the mere thought of characterizing his life as "difficult" sends him scurrying for cover.

What's wrong with "difficulty"? I want to know. I want to redeem it, as both a word and a concept. I want to speak it out loud, without apology, in the same matter-of-fact tone I'd use to say, "I prefer black cats to spotted ones," or "My daughter has been known to eat grasshoppers." And then I want to figure out how I can not merely admit to having a difficult life but also use the difficulties I've acknowledged to enrich the life.

This process requires steering a tricky course between denial to starboard and masochism to port. For social reasons, as I've said, it's tempting to hide from others the fact that you're having a hard time. You want, after all, to appear independent and capable, those most valued traits of the American psyche, or at least, failing that, to be considered a trooper, a good sport. But I don't think this sort of social cover-up is as dangerous as denying your difficulties to yourself. This denial can have nasty bodily consequences for those of us with physical disabilities, as I've learned painfully. Each time I've taken a bad fall, I've been ignoring the limitations fatigue and muscular weakness place on my body. I've been treating my body as though it were some other body, an able body. But it's not. It's mine. A body in trouble. And it's my responsibility to attend to its realities and take proper care of it. I can't do that if I deny that it needs special treatment.

The emotional consequences of denial are subtler and perhaps more devastating. How many times have you been counseled by some well-meaning person, often one who's deep into denying difficulties of her own, "You think too much. You'll only make matters worse. Just ignore the problem, and it will go away"? You have a problem, however, because you are a living being, and thus the problem is inextricably entwined into your life. Ignoring the problem, then, means ignoring some essential element of your life. In some cases, it might "go away" in the sense that the portion of your life into which the problem is woven might atrophy and drop off, like a tree branch strangled by mistletoe. But do you really want a life thus mutilated?

Anyway, the difficulties created by something like MS don't even go away to that extent. Whether you ignore your body or not, you still get tired, your vision blurs, you stumble over a crack in the sidewalk, you wet yourself before you make it to the bathroom, you drop your favorite dish, the one Aunt Elsie gave you before she died, and it smashes to smithereens. The only way you can deny difficulties as mundane and relentless as these— and deny the rage and shame and sadness they produce—

is through emotional anesthesia. You can shut down your feelings. But if you can no longer experience sorrow, how will you experience joy?

"Okay," you say, "you've persuaded me. I'm not going to deny I live a difficult life. I'll freely admit my problems. . . . Wow, have I got problems! Oh, poor me, poor me!" Suddenly there you are, sliding over into that other danger zone I perceived in learning to use difficulty to enhance life. I called it masochism, a taste for suffering for its own sake. Now, an arduous life, well lived, may involve some suffering, but suffering is never its point. Think back to Anne. She didn't go to Zaïre in order to wipe out on a rickety bridge, sending her motorcycle twenty feet straight down into the river while she sprawled, breathless and battered but otherwise intact, thank God, on the splintery boards above. That's what happened, and she bore the bruises for weeks, but that's not the reason she's in Zaïre.

A great pitfall in chronic illness, which often does inflict suffering of some sort, is the temptation to focus on the suffering, even, in a way, to come to live for it. All of us have probably known at least one person—in my case it's an elderly friend with a gallbladder condition—who takes no interest in anything but her own troubles. (Actually, Edna's interest does sometimes extend to the illnesses and deaths of her acquaintances.) This is, indeed, a way of acknowledging life's difficulties, but the route's a dead end which peters out in an isolated swamp of self-pity.

I think there's an authentic alternative to either denial or masochism in response to a difficult life. You can use your hardships to augment your understanding of and appreciation for yourself and the world you dwell in. Because a difficult life is more complicated than an easy one, it offers opportunities for developing a greater range of response to experience: a true generosity of spirit.

One may cry harder in the clutches of a troubled existence, but one may laugh harder as well. I had almost no sense of humor at all, particularly with regard to myself, before I started really experiencing difficulties, in the form of depression and MS. I was as sour as a pickle. Now, my life seems full of merriment. Imagine me, for instance, coming home from a shopping trip one winter evening. As I enter the screened porch, Pinto, my little terrier puppy, bounces forward to greet me, throwing my precarious balance off. I spin around and fall over backward, whacking my head on the sliding glass door to the house, but a quick check (I'm getting good at those) suggests no serious damage this time. This is called a pratfall, a burlesque device used in plays and films for a surefire laugh. In keeping with this spirit, I start to giggle at the image of this woman sprawled flat on her back, helpless under the ecstatic kisses of a spotted mongrel with a comic grin who is thrilled to have someone at last get right down to his own level. The night is chilly. George isn't due home for an hour. Pinto's kisses are unpleasantly damp. "Oh Lord," I think, "if I'm too weak to get up this time, it's going to be a long night." Spurred by the cold and the kisses, I get up.

In addition to making me more humorous, I think the difficult life has made me more attentive. In part, this trait is self-defensive: I *have* to watch out for all kinds of potential threats—bumps and cracks, for instance, and small comic dogs lurking in doorways—that others might ignore without courting disaster. But this is only a drill for a more valuable attentiveness to the objects and people around me. I notice more details. I take more delight in them. I feel much more connected to others than I used to, more aware of their troubles, more tolerant of their shortcomings. Hardship can be terrifically humanizing.

The most valuable response I've developed, I think, is gratitude. I don't mean that I'm grateful for having MS. I'm not, not in the least, and I don't see why I should be. What I'm grateful for is that, in spite of having MS, I've fulfilled ambitions I never dreamed I would. When I was first diagnosed, I didn't think I'd see my children grow up, and now I have a foster son in the navy, a daughter in the Peace Corps, and a son in college. I was sure my illness would drive George and me apart, and now we've celebrated our twenty-fifth wedding anniversary. I couldn't imagine that I'd make it through graduate school, but I did—twice. I thought I'd have to give up on being a writer, but here I am, writing for my life. I might have managed all these things—maybe even managed them better—without having MS. Who can tell? But through having MS, I've learned to cherish them as I don't think I could have otherwise.

In the past couple of years, my condition has deteriorated steadily. In the face of each new loss, I experience a new rush of panic and anger and sometimes despair. All the same, one morning not long ago, as I was sitting on my porch trying to marshal enough energy to stagger into the house, pull on some clothes, and drive to my studio for a day's writing, I felt, beneath the fatigue and fear of falling that were holding me back, a surge of satisfaction. Looking out at Pinto frolicking with a ball, and beyond him at the paloverde tree beside the drive-way, and beyond it to the Santa Catalina Mountains, flat and bluish in the morning light, I thought, "I'm happier now, like this, than I've ever been before."

That's the joy of doing things the hard way.

⌒ Good Enough Gifts ⌒

We are, on the whole, a society of alarmists and malcontents. Nothing that life sends along ever quite reassures or satisfies us. The person without a car, for instance, thinks not about the wholesome exercise walking gives her, or the pounds of carbon monoxide she is keeping out of our fragile atmosphere by riding the bus, but about her deprivation. So she scrapes together the money for an old blue VW bug and then frets because it isn't a Volvo station wagon. But if she finds a Volvo station wagon she can afford—a 1977, say—then she may pine because she can't afford one of those snazzy red BMW convertibles she sees given away on "Wheel of Fortune." The owner of a red BMW convertible, I suppose, laments the lack of a white Rolls-Royce Corniche with a tan leather top.

I happen to be the owner of that 1977 Volvo sta-

tion wagon. I've had it for three years, and I could probably afford by now to trade it in on a 1980 Volvo station
wagon, but I don't want to. It runs well enough so that
the last time I took it in for a tune-up, the mechanic
declined to fiddle with it. I've spent so many hours in it
that I know the location of every control without looking—the windshield wipers and the turn signal, for example, so that even though they're run by the same lever, I
hardly ever scrub my windshield while I'm trying to
change lanes anymore. I recognize its rattles and moans
and squeals. Of course, I don't know how many miles are
on it, since the odometer was stuck at 65,000 when I
bought it, though I'd be willing to bet it's traveled a good
65,000 more. But do I really need to know how far it's
been? Does one, after all, ask a lady her age?

I keep my car for another reason besides its ser-
viceability and familiarity. I keep it because it says something, to me at least, about contentment. To my parents
it may suggest that I don't care whether or not I'm a
shame for the neighbors. To the neighbors it may reveal
that I haven't done very well in the world by contemporary—that is, material—standards. But, settled into my
life the way it is, it represents my ability to accept what
life offers without fretting that I'm missing out on the
goods, that I'm being cheated, above all that there's something *wrong* with me for not wanting—demanding, going
into debt for—more than I've got.

This elderly Volvo may well be my last car, not
because it's going to last forever, but because I'm not.
Already my weakness and clumsiness make me nervous
about driving, and I can foresee the day, perhaps not very

far in the future, when I no longer feel safe even on the quiet streets I try to stick to. I'm afraid of that day. I've had my own car for many years now, and I'm accustomed to taking off in it whenever I like. It signifies independence for me, a self-determination I can hardly bear to lose. And my husband's independence is at stake, too. Once I can no longer drive, George will have to take me to all the places I can't avoid, like the dentist's office, and run even more stupid errands than he does already, making a mad round of bookstores and photo shops and travel agents and dry cleaners and drugstores. I have a genius for dreaming up stupid errands. So this is more than an old car with a dent in the passenger's door and a Peace Corps bumper sticker on the back we're talking about here. This is a way of life.

Ways of life change. No one knows that fact more clearly than the family who lives with multiple sclerosis. They change, and change, and change. Just when you get used to things as they are right now—seeing double, for instance, or having a mother who walks with a cane—a new event throws you off balance and you have to start adjusting all over again, suffering vertigo along with your double vision, maybe, or having a mother in a wheelchair. And most of us don't like change. I hate it so much that I eat the same breakfast of fruit juice and cereal every morning, just so as to start the day feeling sure of something. All changes, even those for the good, make us feel disoriented, fearful of the unknown, out of control. And let's be frank. With MS, changes are all too seldom for the good.

I think it's the fear triggered by change which

causes people to think that the diagnosis of MS cries doom, both for the person who has the disease and for those who care for her or him. I used to teach medical students how to give neurological exams, and I recall clearly one young man who had seen a patient with MS that morning. The patient didn't know, and the doctor this medical student was working with didn't want to tell her, because he thought the diagnosis much too horrible to burden anyone with. What should be done? the medical student asked me. I couldn't give a specific answer, of course. Each patient has individual needs and capacities, and I'd never met this one. But as a general principle, I told the medical student, once you know your patient, you should tell her the truth. Most people I know deal remarkably well with the diagnosis of MS. Most, like me, are relieved to have at least a name for the set of symptoms that may have made them feel lazy or clumsy, if not downright crazy. The person with the problem, in the situation described by the medical student, was not the patient but the doctor. *He* was the one too horrified by the diagnosis to speak of it. And I don't think it's fair to make patients bear their doctors' problems.

This anecdote illustrates an all-too-common approach by those in the "helping" professions—that is, doctors, but also nurses, social workers, psychologists, vocational counselors, and the like. These people are generally physically fit themselves, and they seldom live with people who are chronically ill. Moreover, they have been trained to search out, diagnose, *and then relieve or cure* problems. Thus, when they encounter a person with MS, and often that person's family as well, they immediately assume that this cluster of people is in trouble and that "being in trouble" is always a bad way to be.

I don't want to denigrate people in the helping professions. I admire my brilliant neurologist; I literally owe my life to my supportive psychotherapist; and I respect the urge to love and heal which drives most helpers. All I'm trying to say is that they are trained to look at the world in a particular way—as a structure of problems and solutions—and that their view may not be the most useful one to an MS person and her or his family. The assumption that MS is bad for the family ignores the possibility that MS may also be, in a variety of ways, good for the family; and the helper who tries to intervene in the family's dynamics, assuming that they must be "sick" in some way, risks damaging whatever wholesome processes may be going on. How does the saying go? If it ain't broke, don't fix it. Like my Volvo's mechanic, a helper may need to know how to do an expert tune-up but also when to leave a smoothly running engine alone.

I also don't want to suggest that I think having MS is a good thing. I have been coping with it for about seventeen years now, and I've found only two good points about it: first, it seems to offer some protection from the common cold; and second, it apparently keeps you looking youthful. In view of all the bad consequences it leads to—falls on the head and broken crockery and wet pants and the kind of fatigue that leaves you literally weeping—these advantages are not worth the price. *Having MS is a very bad thing.*

But since there's nothing anyone can do to make it go away, I'm going to stop talking about how bad it is.

There's just no point. Instead, I'm going to consider it a given in some people's lives. Now, our lives are stories we tell ourselves. And they tend to follow, as closely as we can make them, the conventions we have learned from reading (and nowadays watching television and films, too). We want them to contain all the features we've been told belong in a good story: a handsome prince or a beautiful princess, a scary monster who's not quite strong enough to withstand the handsome prince, an ending in which all the evil people are dead or at least in jail and all the good people live happily ever after. True, nowadays the prince may be named Sonny and the monster may be a Miami drug kingpin, but the shape of the story is the same.

Stories of family life also follow predictable lines, as television comedies from "Leave It to Beaver" and "Father Knows Best" to "The Cosby Show" and "Family Ties" illustrate. In each episode, some member of the family develops a problem and, in no more than half an hour's time, with the affectionate and good-humored support of the other family members, resolves the problem to everyone's satisfaction. Next week another problem will arise, of course, but it will be a different problem and it, too, will be resolved before the episode ends. No show depicts the same problem week after week after week. The audience would get bored and switch to another channel. And no problem is ever too tough for the family to lick once and for all if they just try hard enough.

It is difficult, I think, to reject these conventional narratives, which we have learned by heart, which comfort us with their predictability. But if we want to lead authentically healthy lives, we have to let them go. Because believing them can damage our feelings toward ourselves and one another. They do not reveal to us the truth about our lives, and they lead us to expect impossible outcomes. Suppose you're a man who gets MS, for instance. You've grown up with the heroic myth, and its elements seem to fit your situation: you're the hero and MS is the villain. All you have to do is fight MS until it surrenders, vanquished, at your feet, and then you (and the beautiful princess, if you love one, and your children, if you have them) can live happily ever after. Only MS turns out to be very different from a dragon or a drug kingpin. No matter how hard you struggle, it is unconquerable. You are defeated, disgraced; and the beautiful princess and the children stare at you with dark and disappointed eyes. Or suppose you live in a family with a mother who has MS. The problem doesn't change from week to week, it never gets resolved, and you can't even switch the channel when you're bored.

This kind of disillusionment is bound to result if you try to fit your life to the shape of a conventional tale. With or without MS, real life simply doesn't work the same way. To create a book or a television show, you have to cut and condense, leaving out all the tedious parts like who ate what for breakfast, and later lunch, and dinner later still, and choosing just one problem to stand in for all the problems you don't have room to mention. The story you tell yourself in creating a life follows different rules, forcing you to keep details you'd just as soon leave out, like the fact that a zit bursts out on the end of your nose the night before your junior prom. It's very hard to be a beautiful princess with a zit on the end of your nose. What can you do? Well, you can call your date (who might be a handsome prince who never, ever gets zits, but probably he isn't) and tell him you've come down with yellow fever and the doctor has put you in quarantine for at least a week so you won't be able to make the prom after all. Or you can transform yourself into an ordinary girl and go to the prom anyway, wearing a lot of makeup on the end of your nose.

This is the important point about the stories we tell ourselves about our lives: We make them up as we go along. Instead of accepting someone else's tales about princes and monsters and omniscient daddies, we come up with fresh material. We get to choose how the story goes. We can't select every event and detail, of course. We can't decide, for instance, whether or not someone gets MS. MS just *happens.* But—and this is the exciting part— we can choose how we will respond to that happening, what kind of role we will give it in the story we're making up as we go along.

You may choose to view your life as the saddest story ever told and yourself—whether you have MS or love someone who has MS—as a tragic figure in its center. You really may. You're in absolute charge here. I know people who have made that choice. But, to be truthful, I don't know many, either because I tend to avoid such people or, more likely, because there aren't an awful lot of them. Most people who live with MS are looking for ways to spin out tales about love and strength and accomplishment. When a well-meaning friend comes up to one of them and says, "Oh, you poor thing, I just don't know

124

how you manage. You're so brave," most glance over their shoulders to see who's being spoken to. If a counselor rushes up and exclaims, "Oh, how unhappy your family must be," a lot may reply, "If I try to serve my family liver for dinner, they are very, very unhappy. The rest of the time, they're a relatively cheerful bunch."

I may sound as though I'm trivializing the complex pain that MS introduces into family life. That's not my intention at all. What I'm trying to do is *normalize* that pain, making it seem not rare and tragic but natural and manageable. Of course you feel pain if you or someone you love has MS, pain made up of sorrow and anxiety and anger and discouragement. But pain is not necessarily a sign of trouble. In this case, it's simply an appropriate response, indicating emotional health. And the presence of pain in a family doesn't have to mean that the family's in trouble, disintegrating under the pressures of living with chronic illness, ready to fall apart at any moment. That's one possible story. But there are plenty of others.

Here's one. The father is a schoolteacher, a slender, quiet, kind man who keeps himself at a slight emotional distance from the rest of the family. The oldest child, silent and dark, is a foster son who joined the family as a teenager. Now thirty and a petty officer in the navy, he has a wife and two half-grown boys himself. The daughter, small but sturdy, envelops those around her in a whirlwind of motion and emotion. In a little village called Mfuatu in Zaïre, she teaches farmers how to build ponds and grow fish to feed their families. The son is growing out of a sullen and rebellious adolescence into an adulthood dedicated to music. As a college student, he plays

bass in several rock bands and in the Tucson Philhar-
monia.

Oh, yes, in this story the father's wife has MS. The
children's mother has MS. And I—the one with the MS
here—have often felt guilty about my role in their lives,
as though my condition automatically transformed me
into a bad wife and mother, as though my presence
among them could bring them only deprivation and misery. And, to be honest with you, I think I really have
made them feel deprived and miserable at times, more
times than I would wish. But I might have done so even
without MS. People who live for a long time together,
bound closely by love, inevitably disappoint and hurt, as
well as gratify and please, one another.

MS may simply have served, more often than not,
as a handy hook to hang our disappointments and pains
on. I'm thinking of a time, a few years back, when we
were in a lot of trouble as a family. Matthew was acting
out most of this trouble, ditching school and failing
courses and making some pretty creepy friends, and we'd
found a counselor to meet with him individually and also
with all of us together. One afternoon when I was sick,
George, Anne, and Matthew went to a counseling session
without me and spent the whole time, I later found out,
talking about me and the problems my MS caused.

I was angry at the time. I thought they were using
my MS as a scapegoat for all the problems of their own
they refused to acknowledge and deal with. In fact, I still
think so, but I don't feel angry anymore. I see now that
sometimes people feel generally bad about themselves
and their lives, as Matthew obviously did, without ever

quite knowing why. Not every problem has a name and a solution. When my family projected their bad feelings, and the helplessness they felt to understand or stop those feelings, onto my MS, they were providing themselves some much-needed focus. Here was something real, clear, definite, something they hated, something they could struggle with and defy and perhaps even come to terms with one day.

Gradually, in the years since this incident, I've begun to forgive myself for having MS and to stop feeling sorry for my family for having the terrible luck to get stuck with me. I've learned to accept from them the help I wish I didn't need. Long ago, the first summer after I knew I had MS, we hiked down to the bottom of Canyon de Chelly and out again. With the children larking around us, sometimes in front and sometimes behind, George had hold of my elbow every step of the trail, and toward the end he had to haul me back up to the rim like a sack that had sprouted wayward feet. That early hike provided the model for my journey through all the following years. At first, I walked with the aid of a cane, and then of a brace as well; now, except for unsteady steps around the house, I don't walk at all. When I fall, I can no longer pull myself up. I need help with the simplest tasks: tying my shoe-laces, unscrewing a jar lid, putting a book back on the shelf. More important, I need encouragement to get me through the fits of fear and anger and disgust at my own uselessness, reminding me that in some form these are ordinary elements in human existence, not much fun but, as my children would say, no big deal.

This kind of assistance is a lot to demand of a

husband and children, and sometimes friends and other family members as well, all of whom have their own strenuous lives to get on with. Living in a society that values self-sufficiency above every other character trait, and in the age of the Superwoman Syndrome, I've often felt ashamed of my shortcomings, especially as a mother. (I'll bet this would be true even if I didn't have MS. Most women can find something to feel ashamed of.) As I grew too weak and exhausted to keep house, I shifted more and more chores onto Ron and Anne and Matthew. While other children were off taking ballet lessons or cruising the malls with their friends, each of mine in turn learned to wash dishes, push the wheezy old vacuum cleaner, hang and fold laundry, function as my sous-chef in the kitchen. I won't say they performed these tasks eagerly, or even cheerfully, but neither did they complain. They simply carried on, in fits and starts, the business of grow-ing up: taciturn Ron, struggling for the intellectual and emotional development his disrupted life had delayed; Anne the self-willed achiever, gifted with both affection and wit, who made her life seem easier than she often found it; and Matthew with his odd mix of truculence and courtliness, clomping through life in his combat boots, chains and padlocks jangling, ten-inch Mohawk shel-lacked and striped yellow and red.

Years later, when I asked Ron how he had felt having a mother with MS, he shrugged: "I didn't think that much about it. You were just you." And it's true that they seemed to pay no more attention to me than other children did to their mothers, even when I behaved in bizarre ways. One night, I recall, as I walked from the kitchen into the dining room, where Anne was standing with her date, our black cat Eclipse slithered in front of me. His heavy body catching me at the ankles, I pitched forward and crashed to the floor. Anne ran over to dust me off and set me back on my feet, looking concerned but unembarrassed. And Andrew continued to court her for a long while afterward, so I guess my lurching around didn't scare him off, though Anne might have wished it had, since she found him longer on persistence than charm.

All the same, I felt sorry for the children of such a mother. Then, inadvertently, Anne herself released me from my pity and shame. Toward the end of her senior year in college, as she was propelling my stumbling feet toward a shoe store (where she was going to cajole me into buying her a pair of bright blue flats by pledging to love me for*ever,* though I didn't yet know that), I said, "I'm really glad you're so grown-up now that I don't have to worry the way I used to about how humiliated you feel being seen with me in public."

"I never did, you know," she said matter-of-factly, leading me in the direction of the blue flats. "Feel humiliated, that is." *No, I didn't know,* I went on, continuing our conversation in my head as I often do. *I just always assumed that during those exquisitely self-conscious adolescent years, all three of you children in turn cringed whenever we went out together or you brought friends home. I felt humiliated for you. Which serves me right, I guess, for jumping to conclusions about who you are.*

This offhand exchange threw my life into a new sort of relief. I'd assumed, I suddenly realized, that the intersection of motherhood with multiple sclerosis was wholly negative, that my disease could only make me an even worse mother than I'd have been otherwise. But maybe having me for a mother wasn't such a bad fate after all. Maybe it isn't so terrible to have to learn how to scrub cooked-on egg out of a skillet or when to stir sherry into a Newburg sauce or whether you ought to wash your new blue jeans in hot water with your white crew socks. Maybe my children are no more pitiable for having grown up with a crippled mother than I am for being crippled in the first place.

Maybe, just maybe, my companionship and affection have compensated, at least in part, for the burdens MS has placed on us all. Like any mother, I've bandaged broken skin and consoled broken hearts and, as Matthew recalls, I was the one who taught him to waltz, even if he did learn to do it with a limp. And maybe, George reminds me as I write, we're all a little wiser, not merely sadder and tireder, for having lived this way. We've learned—in the teeth of all the romantic novels and television sitcoms and glossy advertising to the contrary—that the bodies we inhabit and the lives those bodies carry on need not be perfect to have value. Bad things *do* happen, we know—to bad and good people alike—but so do good things. Life's curses, like life's blessings, are always mixed.

Increasingly, as I've learned to relax and let reflections of this kind seep in around my worry and guilt, I'm able to accept myself as what Bruno Bettelheim calls a "good enough mother," weariness and shaky legs and feeble fingers and all. The children themselves—the radioman, the Peace Corps volunteer, the symphony musician—unwittingly press me to acceptance. With children this good, what mother, with or without multiple sclerosis, wouldn't feel good enough?

Instead of flagellating myself, I've taken to thinking in terms of the advantages a family with a chronic illness in their midst might find in their circumstances. One is coherence. In our society, grounded in the principles of independence and self-sufficiency, families tend to fragment readily. Many, for instance, are affluent enough to afford each member her or his own television with VCR, stereo, telephone line, even refrigerator and microwave, so that family members don't have to talk to one another even long enough to negotiate whether they'll watch "War and Remembrance" on Channel 4 or "The Frugal Gourmet" on Channel 6. Anyway, on a typical day, Sister's got a track meet at a school across town; Brother's at the dress rehearsal of his drama class's spring play; Mom's working late at the office; Dad's stuck in traffic out on the interstate on his way home from a conference. When they get home, at separate times, they'll pop frigid yummies out of the freezer and into the microwave and eat them in front of the tube. Thus silenced and separated, families are bound to break down. But the family with MS has at least one concern in common. "Sharing" doesn't mean sharing only the goodies, they learn—an occasional trip to Disneyland, say, or Thanksgiving dinner at Grandma's. Sharing afflictions can create bonds just as strong—in my experience, even stronger.

Another advantage MS can bring is tolerance. Tolerance for one another, of course. Here's a charming anecdote I came across in a recent book review to illustrate what I mean: "After a sleepless night dominated by the squalling of a colicky newborn, a young father found himself standing over the crib with a pillow inches from the baby's face, ready to murder it. 'What's the matter with me?' he wails to his therapist. The therapist asks, 'You didn't do it, did you?' The young father answers, 'No, but I wanted to!' The therapist nods. 'Welcome to parenting.' " Welcome to family life in general, I would add. The presence of MS in a family can be infinitely more irritating than a colicky baby's squalls, and one member is bound to feel murderous toward another—caregiver toward MS person, MS person toward caregiver—a good deal of the time. The point, however, is that *we don't do it.* We learn to accept the presence of troublesome feelings as normal to our human being.

Even more important, however, we can learn to tolerate the presence of adversity in our lives. I remember Anne complaining to me a couple of years ago about a friend's lack of sympathy for people in difficulty—the homeless, the hungry, the disabled. "The trouble is," she said thoughtfully, "that he's never had anything bad happen to him. No one in his family has ever lost a job, or gotten sick, or died. He thinks life is supposed to be easy." A lot of people think life is supposed to be easy. And they get furious and bitter when it betrays their expectations. But thanks to the fact that someone in her family has gotten sick, Anne knows that life is neither easy nor fair, though it can be funny and pleasurable from time to time—more often than not, I think she'd say along with me.

Together with coherence and tolerance, the family with MS can learn responsibility for their own well-

132

being. That squalling newborn wants some power to come along and make its colic vanish *right this very instant,* because it is a helpless infant and every event in its life seems to take place by magic. We all carry within us vestiges of that infantile demand to be rescued instantly from whatever we don't like about our circumstances. But we also learn, with maturity, that magical rescue is impossible. No one is going to rescue us from MS. So, unless we want to spend the rest of our lives writhing and screeching like babies with bellyaches, we'd better find out for ourselves how to live as healthily and contentedly as possible. Here, I think, good counseling can help—not to save us from all our troubles but to explore ways of living responsibly with those troubles without letting them dominate our choices and actions.

These are a few, but by no means all, of the advantages I can think of to the inevitable presence of adversity—whether as MS or in some other form—in our lives. I hope that, now that I've got you started, you're thinking of dozens more. The worst is happening—the worst is always happening—and we're surviving it. Troubles? God knows we have plenty of those. But at random we are dealt, along with our calamities, opportunities: to take care of one another, to practice bravery, to delight in even the tiniest accomplishments and pleasures. And so, since we get to choose how to interpret the events that befall us, why not look on them as gifts?

❧ I'm Afraid. I'm Afraid. I'm Afraid. ❧

*A*n elderly woman of my acquaintance—I'll call her Helen—claims that she would like to travel widely but is afraid of flying "alone." She quails in the face of the grim inevitability that, unable to locate her connecting flight, she'll spend the remainder of her life wandering through the purgatorial stench and neon glare of the tunnel connecting United's B and C terminals at O'Hare. It doesn't do any good to assure her that these days it's impossible, unless you're the president or Donald Trump, to clamber aboard an airplane without at least a hundred ninety other people clambering aboard with you and that airport personnel, not to mention fellow travelers, give directions cheerfully and with remarkable accuracy if asked. The company and guidance of strangers don't count. What she wants is someone who will take her by the hand and lead her through all the steps between "here" and "there" without her having to think about them—someone, that is, who will absolve her of responsibility for herself.

So wholly has Helen yielded to the fear that determines what she "can" and "can't" do that she can't imagine living otherwise. I recall describing to her my daughter's behavior on the night before she left us to spend more than two years with the Peace Corps fisheries program in Zaïre: hunched at the table between her boyfriend and me, she pushed her dinner into random patterns on the plate, looking from one of us to the other and finally wailing: *"I'm so scared!"*

"She *was?*" asked Helen.

"Well, sure, she was terrified," I said. "She was going to *Africa.* If she hadn't been frightened, I'd have thought she had at least one screw loose somewhere."

"I guess that's true." Helen laughed a little, but I could see that she had her doubts about what constitutes loose screws. In her system of thinking, Anne couldn't possibly *both* feel dread *and* go to Africa. The one would preclude the other. To go anyway, fear and all, you'd have to be at least a little crazy.

In a woman like Helen, this attitude is probably not surprising. The daughter of an invalid mother, who for years never left her bed, let alone boarded an airplane, Helen clung to her father until she was married and then darted to her husband's sheltering wing. Ted liked this childlike quality in her, which threw his manliness into relief. A slight, quiet man without much education, he might occupy a modest position out in the world; but in his own home, he was a protective giant. Throughout their long marriage, he mediated between her and the world beyond their home, fostering her certainty that she wasn't brave or clever enough to manage without him. Then he died. In the years since, her own competence has surprised her, I think. She's done everything from hammering her first nail into her dining-room wall to purchasing a new car. She continues, however, to draw the line at traveling alone. Sometimes I wonder if she doesn't think that a solo voyage would be disloyal to Ted's memory. She wants to remain his beloved little girl insofar as she can.

In her seventies, Helen is still physically vigorous; but I think that her situation raises some questions for those of us who are physically disabled, and those who care for us, nonetheless. Confronted by the possibility of performing an act that she fears, no longer able to turn like a child to someone who will automatically take the responsibility for getting her through it, she chooses not to do it at all. To avoid conditions that make us afraid is unquestionably one of life's options. But I think it's a choice that serves us poorly if we want to determine for ourselves the quality of our lives.

I, for one, can really identify with Helen's fear. She says she's afraid of flying alone, but beneath that specific manifestation lies the essential dread of entering unfamiliar circumstances with unknown consequences over which she believes herself to have no control. Looked at in this way, her fear is universal. We all feel it, whether reasonably or unreasonably, about some element(s) of our lives. And perhaps those of us who live with a chronic incurable degenerative disease whose course and outcome are almost entirely unpredictable feel it with particular, and particularly relentless, poignancy.

Over the seventeen years I've known I had MS, I've spent more and more of my life feeling fear. I can no longer take a single step without it, because my shuffling feet may trip and throw me to the ground. I've got a lump of scar tissue above my left eye and three crowned front teeth to prove the possibility. When I drive, I'm afraid of having an accident. On shopping trips and long drives, I'm afraid of wetting myself. When I travel alone far from home, I'm afraid I'll collapse in exhaustion with no one to take care of me. All these anxieties are manifestations of the radical terror that now grounds my life: that my MS is getting demonstrably worse and there's nothing anybody can do to stop it and one day—not some comfortingly distant "one day" but a real day, any day now—I'll be bedridden and unable to take care of even my most basic daily needs.

Fear, like anger or grief or any other "negative" emotion, makes us uncomfortable, and so our first inclination is to get rid of it as quickly as possible. In Helen's case, this is easy enough: all she has to do is stay at home, or find a traveling companion willing to take on the equivalent of a small child for a few hours. If you don't do what you fear, you won't feel all those unpleasant symptoms anxiety triggers: dizziness, constricted throat, queasy stomach, icy hands, thudding heart. . . .

Of course, you may never get anywhere, either. That's the real drawback to making the kind of choice Helen has made, I think. In avoiding the discomfort of fearful feelings, you also eliminate the opportunity for courageous action—what Webster's defines as action "marked by bold resolution in withstanding the dangerous, alarming, or difficult"—and the emotional maturity such action develops. Courage is not, after all, either fearlessness or daredeviltry. On the contrary, it is the capacity to carry out your life in the teeth of fear. As such, it offers scant comfort but invaluable aid in rounding and deepening and shading your life. If you happen to feel fear (and who doesn't?), don't duck it: Use it.

Some of fear's usefulness is purely pragmatic. Fear for my footing and my driving, for instance, produces an attentiveness and a caution I really need. Each time I've fallen, I've been thinking about something besides my feet. You recall the old lampoon of Gerald Ford, that he couldn't walk and chew gum at the same time? Well, if I want to stay upright, I *shouldn't* walk and chew gum at the same time. Fear of falling forces my attention where I need it. (True, thinking about nothing but your feet for moments on end gets very, very boring, but that's a separate problem which belongs in another essay.) Similarly, in driving, the alertness my fear triggers helps prevent tight situations in which my weakness might lead to an accident.

Sometimes fear transcends the utilitarian, leading me to question social mores I've accepted unconsciously. Compared to the two days I spent under observation in the Brotman Medical Center in Los Angeles after I ignored my feet and fell on my head, for instance, wet pants may seem relatively trivial, but in fact the very possibility chills me, and the event itself soaks me in shame. These feelings are an inevitable outcome of the toilet-training process, I suspect; without them little children would feel

no impulse to control bladder and bowels. We even suc-
ceed in imposing them on nonhuman creatures, as anyone
knows who has seen her little dog's ears droop and eyes
roll lugubriously at an offending pool of puppy piddle
under the dining-room table. And in the interests of sani-
tation, such dread and shame are all to the good.

Still, when it comes right down to it, wet pants are
messy, they're a nuisance to change, they're excruciat-
ingly embarrassing, but they are not the end of the world.
They're not even close to the end of the world. You can
sit down right this minute and list off the top of your head
at least two dozen things that are much more catastrophic
than wet pants. (The destruction of tropical rain forests
is a good place to start.) If anything, they provide a good
opportunity for setting your social priorities straight. I've
known MS people who refuse to leave their homes for
fear of wetting themselves, but I think they're mixed up
about what really matters. Getting out into the world and
making yourself a place there are important. Staying dry
is important, too—just not as important. So I put on an
incontinence pad, scope out the bathroom first thing no
matter where I am, and hope for the best. Which I sometimes get.

If fear can lead you to figure out what doesn't
really matter, it can also reveal what does. Since the sen-
sations aroused by fear are disagreeable, even painful,
only a masochist would seek them out by performing a
frightful act she doesn't really care about. For me, even
the simple act of leaving the house is risky. I've suffered
from agoraphobia for more than half my life now, and
although the symptoms have abated over the years, I'm

still subject, without warning, to powerful panic attacks that leave me giddy and sick and chilled. For this reason, I'm afraid to travel away from home. And yet I do so, time and again. Travel is part of my life as a writer. It helps me to support myself, and it allows me to interact with audiences so that I don't feel as though I'm working in a vacuum. It forces me into touch with the world, where I gain the experiences I need for writing. I care so much about my work that I dare the damned panic attacks. I wouldn't do the same for deep-sea diving or drag racing or running for public office, for instance, even if I had the requisite stamina and skills. I don't care enough for them. I guess that's how I know I'm a writer: I'll do whatever I have to for it.

The grand test of my traveling mettle is almost upon me. I'm going to Zaïre with my husband to spend Christmas with our daughter. And I've never been scareder in my life. I imagine myself helpless in a world without toilets, much less grab bars, without sidewalks, much less curb cuts. I fantasize that, separated somehow from George and Anne, I'll be arrested in a corrupt dictatorship without habeas corpus where I don't even speak the language. I meditate on the deadly diseases teeming in a single drop of the water Anne carries up from the river for her daily use. I choke on the thought of grasshoppers and palm grubs for dinner, though not of termites, which Anne reports are delicious. I visualize boomslangs slithering through the long grass at the edge of her bare yard. One of the great things I find about fear is the richness of imagination it releases! All the same, I'm going. When the time comes, George may have to carry me aboard the plane babbling and senseless with terror, but by God I'm going to see my daughter and taste the strange life she's chosen (even the palm grubs, if necessary). Because going *matters.*

And if he has to, George will carry me aboard. I trust him to do that. He is just the sort of caregiver a fearful person needs: not a protector, like Helen's father and husband, who in standing between her and her fears prevented her from confronting and braving them, but an encourager, one who gives heart for terrifying leaps into the unknown. He doesn't say, "Don't be afraid." He knows such an instruction is not merely ineffectual but downright harmful, subtly belittling a person's emotional reality. "You're afraid," he says. "That's okay. You can do what you need to anyway."

This is a hard sort of care to give, I think. For one thing, it requires the caregiver to relinquish any pretense of control over another person's life. He may want, with the kindest of motives, to take charge and arrange matters so that the person he cares for will never feel nervous or alarmed, but he must not. Instead of saying, "What a good chance to share your work with new people," leaving me to decide how much that work matters to me, George could say at the start of each trip, "Oh, you don't need to go. All the fretting will just tire you out. Better stay here at home." But he knows that my fear is my own, just as his feelings are his. I'm entitled to it and to the choices it challenges me to make.

For another thing, this kind of care does not preclude suffering, as a more protective form might. As I've said before, fear *hurts,* and the distress sometimes goes on

142

throughout whatever frightening task you've decided to undertake anyway. (In my experience, by the way, it dissipates as soon as the act is finished and is generally followed by a pleasurable flood of fulfillment I don't feel at any other time.) It's a hardy caregiver who doesn't rush in, sticking on emotional Band-Aids right and left and thus preventing you from winning through to your own achievement. The gifted caregiver accepts suffering as natural, often unavoidable, even at times constructive. He provides you reassuring pats and sympathetic kisses and maybe sometimes a bunch of congratulatory posies, but he holds off on the Band-Aids, figuring that time and fresh air heal most of the world's woes.

No matter how much encouragement you receive, however, you're the only one who can cope with your own fear. To do so, you must acknowledge it, but fear is hard to own up to nowadays, I think. Not perhaps for a woman of Helen's generation, for whom timorousness was a desirable feminine trait. In addition to her fear of flying, Helen claims a raft of other socially acceptable phobias—of heights, of thunderstorms, of snakes and mice—which prove her womanly delicacy in contrast to the manly ruggedness of her protectors. But, as "manly ruggedness" suggests, acknowledging fear has never been acceptable behavior in men, even in quite young boys; "You girl!" they snarl at each other's timidity, the unkindest cut of all. And one of the least constructive consequences of the women's movement has been the belief of many women that the way to achieve equality lies in adopting male values and behaviors. Thus, virtually all of us have come to view our fears with shame and to disguise them from others under a show of toughness or insouciance. We substitute *bravado,* "showy . . . conduct . . . often characterized by bluster and swagger," for *bravery,* the ability to "meet danger or endure pain or hardship without giving in to fear." Note that the definition of *bravery* does not say "without fear." On the contrary, the presence of fear is intrinsic to it: you must feel the fear in order to resist and refuse it.

Well, but what's wrong with pretending you don't feel fear? After all, by *pretending* you're not afraid, maybe you'll stop *being* afraid. Maybe . . . but I doubt it. Fear, like those other "negative" emotions, anger and grief and so on, which society teaches us to repress, survives beneath the level of pretense, and refusing to admit to it can actually strengthen it. As linguists and anthropologists know, the act of naming an entity grants the namer power over the named. What we refuse to utter flourishes out of psychological reach; what we can articulate, we can control. By attaching shame to certain basic human emotions, social rules prohibit us from speaking aloud about some of the strongest and most painful areas of our lives. And in our silence, cut off from one another, cut off sometimes even from our own feelings, too ashamed to admit that we quake and rage and sob inside, we lose the chance to take full charge of our selves.

Fear and anger and grief feel so unpleasant to us that we're eager to transform them into confidence and affection and joy. But you can't transform what you haven't grasped. The first step toward transformation is to locate your feelings, recognize them, admit them out loud to yourself and, when necessary, to others. This is risky, I know. You may communicate ideas you've been taught aren't "nice" to talk about. (How horrified a woman like Helen would be, for example, by my speaking to you about wet pants! Ladies do not refer to bodily functions in public.) That's all right. Plenty of people have thought they'd die of embarrassment, but no one has actually done it. And by naming your "shameful" feelings, you take possession over them instead of letting them possess you. This is the beginning of transformative power.

And so I say, *I'm afraid of having MS: of the almost daily deterioration of my strength; of the loss of control over my own body; of my increasing dependence on others to help me with the simplest personal tasks—tying my shoes, getting out of bed. Where will it all end? I'm afraid. I'm afraid. I'm afraid.* But like other MS people (and on the whole we're not very different from people in general, except perhaps that our fears are more focused and therefore easier to get at if we try), I don't give in to my fears. *If I weren't scared of this catastrophic disease,* I remind myself, *I'd have at least one screw loose somewhere.* So I put my fears to the best use I can, analyzing them to discover how to live carefully and choose my actions wisely. I'm nourished by the encouragement of others, like George, who believe that what's important is not that I'm scared but that I do what I need to do whether I'm scared or not. By speaking my fear aloud, I've reduced it from a giant trampling my interior landscape to an ordinary imp, the kind who dances through everybody's inner house from time to time, curdling the milk and smashing the crockery but leaving the structure basically intact. Surveying the damage, I get out my mop and broom. *This is my life,* I say to myself, *fear and all. I'm responsible for it. And I'd better get on with it, because it matters.*

Where I Never Dreamed I'd Go, and What I Did There

Not long before my husband and I are scheduled to embark for a two-week visit to our daughter, a Peace Corps volunteer in Zaïre, Anne is summoned to Kinshasa, the capital of the country, by the local representative of Lufthansa Airlines. This demand is decidedly easier made than met, entailing as it does shortwave and hand-carried communications followed by a journey of a couple of hundred kilometers, part of it on a Yamaha 125 motorcycle over the slippery ruts of dirt roads in rainy season. Nonetheless, Anne reaches the city and presents herself at the Lufthansa office.

We learn about her visit a couple of weeks later. Getting a message, via the network of Peace Corps parents that crisscrosses this country, to call Anne on Saturday at midnight, George and I take turns dialing; and after an hour we hear the characteristic chirp of her "Hello," as clear as though she were still at college in Massachusetts and not on the other side of the world. The Lufthansa representative wanted to tell her, she reports, that he'd received word that her handicapped mother was coming but the airline would not risk the liability of providing any assistance. There were no Jetways. Could her mother walk down the stairs?

"Well, I guess she'll have to," Anne says she told him.

"Well, I guess I'll have to," I echo, in as offhand a tone as I can muster while trying to imagine how many steps are required to connect the door of a DC-10 to the ground. Many, I decide.

There is one wheelchair at the airport, she was told, but the representative couldn't guarantee that it would be available. Her mother would have to walk from the plane to the terminal.

"Tell him," I say, out of breath from mentally descending all those stairs and not at all ready to cross a gulf of tarmac, "that I'm bringing my own wheelchair. Tell him I want it unloaded and brought to me at the plane." Does one really tell a Lufthansa representative this sort of thing? I wonder. Does a Lufthansa representative listen?

"He ended up," Anne says at last, "by asking, 'Do your parents know what they're doing? Are they sure they really want to come here?' I said yes. I told him you really want to come."

Actually, by this point in our conversation, I have to confess, I'm not at all as sure as she made me sound. George and I have never traveled abroad before, and Africa

148

certainly doesn't sound like the best choice for a shake-down cruise. But it seems much too late for second thoughts. We have our passports, our visas, our tickets and hotel reservations. We've gotten typhoid, tetanus, yellow fever, cholera, and gamma globulin shots, as well as anti-malarial drugs. Our duffel bags are half-packed with a weird assortment of Anne's requests—everything from little toys for the children in her village and hairball medication for her cats to the flavor packets from Kraft Macaroni & Cheese Dinners. More persuasive than anything else, however, is the sound of her voice in my ear. Since she left more than a year ago, we've had a series of thrilling letters, several dozen snapshots, one tape recording, and one other telephone call. I have not looked into her eyes in all that time. I have not once put my arms around her. The Lufthansa representative is going to have to come up with more than a flight of stairs and a sea of tarmac to dissuade me from spending Christmas with my daughter.

"Sure we're sure," I hear George say over the extension in the living room. "We'll manage." That's what he always says. And he always makes it come true.

On Christmas Eve, we begin our descent into Kinshasa just as the moon rises, enormous, orange, barred by thin purple-gray clouds, a perfect African moon. For a long moment, its exotic light distracts me from my growing terror of the ordeal to come: the steps, the tarmac, images of myself stumbling and tumbling down, down, down. I'm tired. We've traveled more than ten hours today, and yesterday as well. What if my legs, weak even when I'm rested, refuse to hold me at all? What if I freeze at the top

149

of the stairs, or sink to the ground in a faint? I don't know. I can't think of any answers. I'll just have to wait to find out.

After the other passengers have left, George and I head for the door. There, we are greeted by the selfsame Lufthansa representative. I'd imagined a tall, stocky man, iron-haired and dour, but instead he's slim and cheerful, a young Belgian who lived for years in Los Angeles and is about to move back there. He's leaving that very evening. When he tells us that, his feet nearly tap-dance with delight. "Your daughter is waiting for you," he says, gesturing out into the warm, sticky darkness.

I look down the flight of stairs. It is very long. My wheelchair, sitting already at the bottom, looks like a toy to me. With my good right hand on the railing, George's hand gripping my elbow, the young Lufthansa representative directly in front, half-turned, ready to break my fall, I inch forward. One, I say to myself. Two. I'm doing it. The ground is getting closer. The wheelchair is growing to ordinary size. I'm there. I'm in it. George is wheeling me a long way across the tarmac into the terminal. I could never have walked such a distance, I think. But of course I don't know that for sure. "You never know what you can do until you have to do it," I routinely tell people who exclaim that they could never cope with MS the way I do. Now I'm putting my platitude to the test.

The young man leads us to the VIP Lounge and turns us over to Mulamba, the Peace Corps faciliteur, whom Anne has asked to meet us and guide us through customs. He greets us gravely and, almost without a word, disappears with our passports and baggage checks.

Before very long he returns and beckons: "Come." We follow him into a large, bare rotunda. Suddenly, in a whirl of bright cotton, pale hair, ruddy skin, Anne rushes through an archway into our arms.

Chez Corps de la Paix sits on a hillside in Mbanza-Ngungu, a city of about thirty thousand in the region of Bas-Zaïre. The house, built by Belgian colonials, is graceful and spacious though crumbling now in the relentless damp. The volunteers from throughout the region have gathered for a slightly belated Christmas fête. Most of them live alone at their posts, coming into Mbanza-Ngungu once every three months to overhaul their motorcycles, to withdraw increasingly worthless zaïres from the bank, and to stock up on cases of staples like sardines and rosy toilet paper with the texture and absorbency of crêpe paper.

This is the only time most of them have the chance to speak English, and from the din around me, I'd say that they're trying to cram three months' worth of repressed speech into a few hours. Since the floors are tile and the house is built on two levels, I can't move around on my own, so I spend most of my time in a corner of the couch, awash in surges of language, of laughter, of rock music from the tape recorder beside me, of thunder crashing from hill to hill around us. Now and then the cooking contingent consults me as they approximate a traditional American Christmas feast: scrawny chickens flown in frozen from South Africa, dressing, potatoes and gravy, green beans, salad, and balls of ground squash seeds called mbika, with chocolate chip cookies for dessert.

They've even found some cream, and George is concocting a potent if immature eggnog.

Anne asked me to bring some copies of *Plaintext* for her to give to her friends, and these are scattered around. A young man comes to me carrying one, open, his finger pointing to a sentence I wrote a good half-dozen years ago: "I'll never make it to Tibet."

"I don't believe this," he tells me gravely. I look at him, at the volunteers swirling around the room in their bright pagnes and boubous, at the crotons higher than a man's head outside the open door. I have to laugh. I still don't think I'll make it to Tibet. But I wouldn't swear.

In Africa, we are an event. "Mundele! Mundele!" children shout, waving and running alongside the battered yellow Peugeot taxi we've hired, as we drive through their villages. *White person! White person!* Whenever we stop, they crowd against the windows, their eyes wide, murmuring and giggling. "Mbote," Anne has taught us to say to them, shaking as many hands as we can reach.

While I get out of the car and slowly pull myself upright on my cane, Edouard, our chauffeur's young apprentice, pulls the wheelchair out of the back, unfolds it, and seats me in it. This is a novelty even greater than our mere presence: a mundele under a gray straw hat bumping and jouncing across the ground in a padded aluminum chair with little wheels on the bottom. There must be crippled Zaïroises. In a Third World country like this, where poverty and disease are elements of daily life for all but a handful of the most privileged (and most corrupt) citizens, where a baby's birth is not celebrated because her chances for survival are slender, where a person may break a leg or be bitten by a cobra hundreds of kilometers from the nearest medical aid, surely physical impairment must be common. But in our brief stay we don't have time to find out what becomes of the physically disabled. We see some people carrying sticks they seem to use as canes or crutches, but never another wheelchair.

In Africa, people stare at oddities. I like that, I find. In the States, people are always averting their eyes. Little children often gaze and point at me, especially if I'm in my electric cart, which must look to them like something escaped from a carnival ride; but their parents hiss and tug them away. They're only trying to teach them "manners," of course, in a society in which a gaze symbolizes an assault. But the consequence of this custom is that I feel invisibilized, if there were such a word; negated; disappeared, to use the term Latin America has given us. "If I can't see you," the eyes sliding uneasily away from my body tell me, "you can't be you." Not *you,* that is, *the way you really are:* lurching along on a cane or hunched in a wheelchair, with curled-up hands and skinny stick legs. I feel, when someone looks away like this, too awful to contemplate. Myself, I'd rather feel like an event.

Maybe other people, when they plan a trip into the unknown, imagine the glorious scenery they'll see or the exotic foods they'll sample or the novel art forms they'll discover. I think about these things too, a little bit, but mostly I think about bathrooms. Or, in the case of Zaïre, the absence of bathrooms. In Kinshasa, and also in

Mbanza-Ngungu, we find flush toilets; and, except for one night during a heavy rainstorm, which Anne says always disrupts water service, these work. En brousse, however, where there's neither electricity nor running water, we know we'll have only waysays. A waysay is a small hut, generally built of wattle and daub and thatched with palm fronds, with a deep hole in the center of the log or earth floor, over which one squats. Not, however, *this* one. The squatting days of this one ended about a decade ago.

With this deficiency in mind, I've stuffed the duffel bags with incontinence shields. We even found a portable potty, really just a campstool with a toilet seat to which a plastic bag can be attached, lightweight and compact enough to fit in the baggage, and this comes in handy more than once. Anne has given the matter plenty of forethought, as well, commissioning a local carpenter to create for her waysay a chair with a hole in the seat. And what a creation! An armchair the size of a modest throne, built of sturdy planks, the rear part of the seat hinged to create an opening above the waysay hole. The seat is so broad that I have to inch myself back across it until I reach the opening. Anne, being in fine physical condition, simply launches herself backward through the air. This structure is too wide for the waysay door, so the carpenter knocks down the wall, leaving one side of the hut completely open. No matter. The waysay faces dense forest, and nobody's likely to peer in but the goats and chickens that forage there.

In spite of these careful preparations, occasionally I find myself in a village away from home needing to use a waysay. The local rules of modesty forbid George from accompanying me, but Anne has been taking care of me almost as long as he has. With her coaching, I manage to straddle the hole and avoid my tennis shoes. "Quelle victoire!" I record in my journal. It's really true: You never know what you can do until you have to do it.

More than once, while Anne and George hike off with local farmers to inspect the ponds where she is teaching them to grow tilapia, Nile perch, for food, I have to be left behind. I try not to mind. I try not to feel as though I'm being left not "behind" but "out," as though life were going on anywhere but where I am, as though I were missing all the fun. This is not a feeling peculiar to Zaïre. As I grow weaker and can walk fewer and fewer steps, even with help, I often get left behind. And I'm learning to accept this arrangement not as a limitation to but as an alteration of my experience. I'm learning to let whatever happens to me, wherever I am, be enough: watching a group of children sway in the branches of a low tree, shouting and singing "Pensez poisson!" until the tree gives with a *crack!* and they tumble into the grass below; chatting in my limited French with Ma Charlotte in her open-air kitchen as she prepares us a meal of smoked fish and boiled sesame seeds and tough green nsaki and rubbery fufu. But sometimes, as I watch people stride off at will, I grieve for the freedom I've lost.

Perhaps Tata Nlandu, an enterprising Zaïrois in his twenties, one of Anne's most promising candidates, senses this grief. Perhaps that's why he announces, when Tata Nzulu is going to harvest one of his ponds, that I too must see a récolte. He will carry me there himself. And he does, at breakneck speed, down half a mile of steep, slippery hillside. By grasping my left wrist in my right hand, I can keep my arms around his neck. The rest of me is too weak to cling, and so I bounce against his back, as limp as a Matadi flour sack. When he feels me slipping, he stops and bends sharply forward, hitching me higher. The ground lurches up toward my face abruptly, then recedes as he resumes his course, his rubber boots slapping the muddy path. The green world is leaping and jiggling all around me. I can't believe what I'm doing. I can't believe I'm plummeting through the jungle on the back of a man to whom I can say nothing but "mbote": literally, "good." I couldn't ask him to stop if my life depended on it. Which it might. I don't scream once. I mewl every now and then, but I don't actually scream.

In this way, I too am enabled to witness the process that shapes the contours of Anne's new life: the pond site selected and laid out with sticks and string; the pond itself scraped out of the jungle, with only machetes and shovels for tools; the barrage built to dam the stream; the compost heaped in opposite corners to create the bloom of plankton that will feed the little fish. And finally, every six months, this récolte: barrage breached, water drained, fish scooped into buckets and basins to be weighed and then sold to the villagers, pond laboriously reconstructed and then restocked with the fingerlings set aside during the harvest, the whole process beginning again. I've been told about all this, of course. But I'm glad to witness it myself, from the shady hillside where Tata Nlandu deposits me in my wheelchair, carried down by Edouard, under an nsafu tree, like a queen surveying her boggy realm. Firsthand experience has a pungency that no telling, however vividly detailed, can quite match.

What goes down must come up, of course, and generally with greater effort, since gravity can't be reversed, and anyway, the sun has broken through a pearly sky, turning the air steamy. When the fish have all been divided and distributed, including a few leftovers for the dancing children, who stuff their wriggling prizes into their shirt fronts or pockets, the récolte is over. To carry me out, Tata Nlandu takes turns with Tata Vita, the sweet-natured but scrawny secretary of Anne's farmers' group. I feel as though I'm being carried by a skeleton, my bones bouncing against his bones so that my sternum and pelvis will be bruised for several days. And because he's no taller than I, my feet drag on the muddy path or tangle in the weeds on either side. Tata Nlandu takes the final stint and, huffing and heaving, staggers at last out of the forest onto the roadway.

"You never know what you can do," I suppose I might have told Tata Nlandu and Tata Vita if I knew the words in Kikongo, "until you have to do it." Except, of course, that they don't have to do it. They choose to do it, for their own reasons, which without a common language I can't quite figure out: a mixture of affection for Mama Anna, their Fish Volunteer, which they extend readily to Mama Nancy, and pride in the work they've undertaken to feed themselves and their families, and resourcefulness in the face of difficulty.

Les Zaïroises, Anne has told us, are good at making

do. They have to be. In a whole year, one of these farmers may earn no more than the equivalent of $125. What's broken must be fixed, or new uses invented for the broken parts. Most of life's demands necessitate physical labor. Without either telephone or automobile, for instance, the only way to check on the health of the grandchild being treated for meningitis at the hospital in Gombe-Matadi is to walk the forty kilometers there and then walk home again to tell the others the good news: Simba has regained consciousness, he's sipping water, the doctor thinks he may recover. In this context, perhaps Tata Nlandu's reasoning isn't mysterious: If you come upon a woman whose legs don't work, you carry her.

The day before leaving Zaïre, we visit the ivory marché in Kinshasa, a scene to strike terror through the heart of all but the most intrepid cripple. I am not intrepid. In fact, I am very, very trepid. I may undertake a variety of schemes, some more harebrained than others, but I never do so without fear.

Here's the ivory marché: two parallel long, low structures, with roofs but no walls, the sides lined by makeshift wooden tables, a long narrow dirt passageway down the middle. This aisle is not crowded with shoppers, at least today, but the vendeurs cluster around us so thickly that we can barely make our way. Because the ground is uneven and thoroughly scuffed, using the wheelchair seems impossible, so I am on foot. We refuse to look at ivory, but we want to buy malachite. On table after table lie arrays of carved malachite owls and frogs and elephants, malachite and brass bangles, strings of malachite beads.

As we pass them, the vendeurs tug us backward to look at something we've missed, forward to glimpse undreamed-of treasures, side to side to side. . . . Their wares are essentially alike, and so we try to buy something from each one. But of course one can't simply plunk down one's zaïres and walk off with one's merchandise. Il faut discouter la prix. The prices they first quote are outrageous, naturally, though the prices we finally get them down to seem like bargains to us. Maybe they are, and maybe they aren't. We have no way of knowing. But we're pleased enough with what we buy: a lot of malachite and also some marriage money, some Kenya bags, a carved chef's staff decorated with a buffalo tail, three colorful paintings on the backs of Matadi flour sacks.

All our transactions are conducted at top volume. Gradually the shouts, the gesticulations, the bright black faces up against ours, the glint of sunlight from the malachite's violent green, the sheen of brass, the muggy smell of jostling bodies in Kinshasa's riparian heat whirl into a synesthetic kaleidoscope. I've discovered that if I stay with George and Anne, I get shoved and grappled as they do. But if I go on a little by myself, the vendeurs press close but touch me only lightly or not at all. I wonder if they think me, tottering along on my cane, ndoki (a bad spirit). Actually, I suspect they simply realize that if they nudge me, I'll fall over, and then I'll be in no position to buy anything. At any rate, I stagger along in a kind of febrile dream.

At last we all stumble, ears ringing, skin sticky,

mouths parched, out the other end of the marché and make gratefully for our waiting taxi. The others seem just as fagged as I am. The ivory marché is the Great Equalizer, chewing up the energies of crippled and able-bodied alike, spitting us all out, limp and dizzy, into the air-conditioned solitude of our room at l'Hôtel de la Gombe.

We have only just gathered Anne into our arms in the rotunda of the terminal at Kinshasa Airport, it seems, and now we must release her there again. George spins the wheelchair around and pushes me through the gate, across the tarmac, to the waiting jet. Swissair apparently has a different policy toward handicapped passengers, because suddenly I find myself in the air, wheelchair and all, between two strapping mundeles. At a sedate pace, they ascend the steps toward the plane. All the same, my heart is racing. *One slip . . .* , I can't help thinking. Involuntarily, my eyes squeeze shut, but I force them open again.

And so this is my last glimpse of Africa: the dilapidated airport, an Air Zaïre jet a little beyond ours, sunlight glancing from the fronds of feather palms, in the distance Kinshasa's few tall buildings against an opalescent sky, the whole view blurred by tears and swaying gently to the slow, erratic rhythm of the footsteps carrying me carefully up one step after another.

What if I'd never come? I ask myself. *How could I bear never to have seen this?*

And this is the only way I know to live as a woman with multiple sclerosis: not to listen to the ominous questions of Lufthansa agents but to hear instead the confidence (even if you think it's misplaced) of the daughter who believes that you're sure what you want to do, of the husband who says you can manage together, of yourself, in whose pronouncement that "you never know what you can do until you have to do it" hides the stronger, even more enabling message: "If you decide you *have* to do something, you'll do it. And you might be lucky enough to miss your tennis shoes in the process."